Ariel Shidlo, PhD
Michael Schroeder, PsyD
Jack Drescher, MD
Editors

Sexual Conversion Therapy: Ethical, Clinical and Research Perspectives

Sexual Conversion Therapy: Ethical, Clinical and Research Perspectives has been co-published simultaneously as *Journal of Gay & Lesbian Psychotherapy*, Volume 5, Numbers 3/4 2001.

*Pre-publication
REVIEWS,
COMMENTARIES,
EVALUATIONS . . .*

"This important book gives voice to those men and women who have experienced painful, degrading, and unsuccessful conversion therapy and survived. Each article, written by a leading investigator, therapist, or theorist in the field of conversion therapy targeted at lesbian and gay individuals, addresses an important aspect of this complex issue. The effects of poor practice, ethical violation, and ill-informed intention on often-young gay/lesbian individuals looking for help in dealing with awareness of homosexual affections in our society have been well documented here.

This book is a valuable collection of readings on the pseudo science of reparative therapy. It is an invaluable resource for mental health providers and policy makers. Indeed, any individual struggling with understanding the dynamics of gay/lesbian identity development in a homophobic/heterosexist society and faced with pressures to change their sexual orientation would be wise to turn to this book for information and guidance."

Joyce Hunter, DSW
*Research Scientist
HIV Center for Clinical & Behavioral Studies
New York State Psychiatric Institute/
Columbia University
New York City, NY*

"This volume is a vivid personal documentation of the harm that conversion therapy may produce in the lives of gay, lesbian, and bisexual individuals. The message underlying such attempts to 'repair' them is that they cannot adequately deal with their life issues until they are cured of their sexual desires. A theme that runs through the personal accounts of former patients contained in this collection is that individuals who enter conversion therapy are seen as being defective, sick, or sinful, and are likely to end up feeling even more so when they fail to change. Many of these accounts describe what they may be characterized as therapeutic abuse, as when one individual was told that homosexual relationships are not based on love but on hostility. A former patient explained that his therapist's intended good 'did me in fact irreparable harm, which it took me not years but decades to realize fully.' This book is an invaluable resource fior those professionals who wish to do no harm."

Marvin R. Goldfried, PhD
Professor of Psychology
State University of New York
at Stony Brook

"Shidlo, Schroeder, and Drescher's *Sexual Conversion Therapy: Ethical, Clinical and Research Perspectives* should be required reading for all therapists whose clients consider conversion therapy, as well as for researchers, ethicists, and policy makers working in this area. This landmark book draws together diverse perspectives, new research data, and creative thinking, bringing them to bear on a complex controversy that affects so many lives."

Ken Pope, PhD, ABPP
Author
Ethics in Pyschotherapy and Counseling,
Second Edition

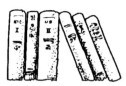

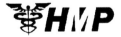

The Haworth Medical Press
An Imprint of The Haworth Press, Inc.

Sexual Conversion Therapy: Ethical, Clinical and Research Perspectives

Sexual Conversion Therapy: Ethical, Clinical and Research Perspectives has been co-published simultaneously as *Journal of Gay & Lesbian Psychotherapy*, Volume 5, Numbers 3/4 2001.

The *Journal of Gay & Lesbian Psychotherapy* Monographic "Separates"

Below is a list of "separates," which in serials librarianship means a special issue simultaneously published as a special journal issue or double-issue *and* as a "separate" hardbound monograph. (This is a format which we also call a "DocuSerial.")

"Separates" are published because specialized libraries or professionals may wish to purchase a specific thematic issue by itself in a format which can be separately cataloged and shelved, as opposed to purchasing the journal on an on-going basis. Faculty members may also more easily consider a "separate" for classroom adoption.

"Separates" are carefully classified separately with the major book jobbers so that the journal tie-in can be noted on new book order slips to avoid duplicate purchasing.

You may wish to visit Haworth's website at . . .

http://www.HaworthPress.com

. . . to search our online catalog for complete tables of contents of these separates and related publications.

You may also call 1-800-HAWORTH (outside US/Canada: 607-722-5857), or Fax: 1-800-895-0582 (outside US/Canada: 607-771-0012), or e-mail at:

getinfo@haworthpressinc.com

Sexual Conversion Therapy: Ethical, Clinical, and Research Perspectives, edited by Ariel Shidlo, PhD, Michael Schroeder, PsyD, and Jack Drescher, MD (Vol. 5, No. 3/4, 2001). *"THIS IS AN IMPORTANT BOOK. . . . AN INVALUABLE RESOURCES FOR MENTAL HEALTH PROVIDERS AND POLICYMAKERS. This book gives voice to those men and women who have experienced painful, degrading, and unsuccessful conversion therapy and survived. The ethics and misuses of conversion therapy practice are well documented, as are the harmful effects." (Joyce Hunter, DSW, Research Scientist, HIV Center for Clinical & Behavioral Studies, New York State Psychiatric Institute/Columbia University, New York City)*

Gay and Lesbian Parenting, edited by Deborah F. Glazer, PhD, and Jack Drescher, MD (Vol. 4, No. 3/4, 2001). *Richly textured, probing. These papers accomplish a rare feat: they explore in a candid, psychologically sophisticated, yet highly readable fashion how parenthood impacts lesbian and gay identity and how these identities affect the experience of parenting. Wonderfully informative. (Martin Stephen Frommer, PhD, Faculty/Supervisor, The Institute for Contemporary Psychotherapy, New York City)*

Addictions in the Gay and Lesbian Community, edited by Jeffrey R. Guss, MD, and Jack Drescher, MD (Vol. 3, No. 3/4, 2000). *Explores the unique clinical considerations involved in addiction treatment for gay men and lesbians, groups that reportedly use and abuse alcohol and substances at higher rates than the general population.*

Sexual Conversion Therapy: Ethical, Clinical and Research Perspectives

Ariel Shidlo, PhD
Michael Schroeder, PsyD
Jack Drescher, MD
Editors

Sexual Conversion Therapy: Ethical, Clinical and Research Perspectives has been co-published simultaneously as *Journal of Gay & Lesbian Psychotherapy*, Volume 5, Numbers 3/4 2001.

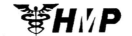

The Haworth Medical Press
An Imprint of
The Haworth Press, Inc.
New York • London • Oxford

Published by

The Haworth Medical Press®, 10 Alice Street, Binghamton, NY 13904-1580 USA

The Haworth Medical Press® is an imprint of The Haworth Press, Inc., 10 Alice Street, Binghamton, NY 13904-1580 USA.

Sexual Conversion Therapy: Ethical, Clinical and Research Perspectives has been co-published simultaneously as *Journal of Gay & Lesbian Psychotherapy*, Volume 5, Numbers 3/4 2001.

Cover design by Jennifer M. Gaska.

Library of Congress Cataloging-in-Publication Data

Sexual conversion therapy: ethical, clinical, and research perspectives / Ariel Shidlo, Michael Schroeder, Jack Drescher, editors.
    p. ; cm.
    "Co-published simultaneously as Journal of gay & lesbian psychotherapy, v. 5, nos. 3/4, 2001."
    Includes bibliographical references and index.
    ISBN 0-7890-1910-8 (hard : alk. paper)–ISBN 0-7890-1911-6 (pbk. : alk. paper)
    1. Homosexuality. 2. Gays–Mental health. 3. Gays–Mental health services. 4. Psychotherapy. I. Shidlo, Ariel. II. Schroeder, Michael PsyD. III. Drescher, Jack, 1951-IV. Journal of gay & lesbian psychotherapy.
    [DNLM: 1. Homosexuality–psychology. 2. Behavior Therapy–methods. 3. Ethics, Clinical. 4. Research. WM 611 S5123 2001]
RC558.S494 2001
616.89′14′08664–dc21
                                                                    2001059452

Indexing, Abstracting & Website/Internet Coverage

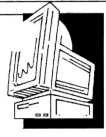

This section provides you with a list of major indexing & abstracting services. That is to say, each service began covering this periodical during the year noted in the right column. Most Websites which are listed below have indicated that they will either post, disseminate, compile, archive, cite or alert their own Website users with research-based content from this work. (This list is as current as the copyright date of this publication.)

Abstracting, Website/Indexing Coverage . . . . Year When Coverage Began

- *Abstracts in Anthropology* 1991
- *Academic Index (on-line)* 1992
- *BUBL Information Service: An Internet-based Information Service for the UK higher education community <URL: http://bubl.ac.uk/>* 1995
- *CNPIEC Reference Guide: Chinese National Directory of Foreign Periodicals* 1995
- *Contemporary Women's Issues* 1998
- *e-psyche, LLC <www.e-psyche.net>* 2000
- *Expanded Academic ASAP <www.galegroup.com>* 1993
- *Expanded Academic Index* 1995
- *Family Studies Database (online and CD/ROM) <www.nisc.com>* 1998
- *Family Violence & Sexual Assault Bulletin* 1992
- *FINDEX <www.publist.com>* 1999
- *Gay & Lesbian Abstracts <www.nisc.com>* 1999
- *GenderWatch <www.slinfo.com>* 1999
- *HOMODOK/"Relevant" Bibliographic database, Documentation Centre for Gay & Lesbian Studies, University of Amsterdam (selective printed abstracts in "Homologie" and bibliographic computer databases covering cultural, historical, social and political aspects of gay & lesbian topics)* 1995

(continued)

- *Index Guide to College Journals (care list compiled by integrating 48 indexes frequently used to support undergraduate programs in small to medium sized libraries)* 1999
- *Index to Periodical Articles Related to Law* 1993
- *InfoTrac Custom <www.galegroup.com>* 1998
- *Leeds Medical Information* 1995
- *MasterFILE: updated database from EBSCO Publishing* 1998
- *MLA International Bibliography (available in print, on CD-ROM and Internet)* 1995
- *Periodcial Abstracts, Research II (broad coverage indexing & abstracting data-base from University Microfilms International (UMI))* 1993
- *Referativnyi Zhurnal (Abstracts Journal of the All-Russian Institute of Scientific and Technical Information-in Russian)* 1991
- *Sage Family Studies Abstracts (SFSA)* 1993
- *Social Services Abstracts <www.csa.com>* 1991
- *Social Work Abstracts* 1993
- *Sociological Abstracts (SA) <www.csa.com>* 1991
- *Studies on Women Abstracts* 1993
- *Violence and Abuse Abstracts: A Review of Current Literature on Interpersonal Violence (VAA)* 1995

Special Bibliographic Notes related to special journal issues (separates) and indexing/abstracting:

- indexing/abstracting services in this list will also cover material in any "separate" that is co-published simultaneously with Haworth's special thematic journal issue or DocuSerial. Indexing/abstracting usually covers material at the article/chapter level.
- monographic co-editions are intended for either non-subscribers or libraries which intend to purchase a second copy for their circulating collections.
- monographic co-editions are reported to all jobbers/wholesalers/approval plans. The source journal is listed as the "series" to assist the prevention of duplicate purchasing in the same manner utilized for books-in-series.
- to facilitate user/access services all indexing/abstracting services are encouraged to utilize the co-indexing entry note indicated at the bottom of the first page of each article/chapter/contribution.
- this is intended to assist a library user of any reference tool (whether print, electronic, online, or CD-ROM) to locate the monographic version if the library has purchased this version but not a subscription to the source journal.
- individual articles/chapters in any Haworth publication are also available through the Haworth Document Delivery Service (HDDS).

Sexual Conversion Therapy: Ethical, Clinical and Research Perspectives

CONTENTS

What Needs Fixing? An Introduction　　1
Ariel Shidlo, PhD
Michael Schroeder, PsyD
Jack Drescher, MD

I'm Your Handyman: A History of Reparative Therapies　　5
Jack Drescher, MD

The View from Irving Bieber's Couch: "Heads I Win,
　Tails You Lose"　　25
Paul Moor

Excerpts from *Cures: A Gay Man's Odyssey*　　37
Martin Duberman, PhD

Becoming Gay: A Personal Odyssey　　51
Richard A. Isay, MD

Healing Homosexuals: A Psychologist's Journey
　Through the Ex-Gay Movement and the Pseudo-Science
　of Reparative Therapy　　69
Jeffry G. Ford, MA, LP

Cures versus Choices: Agendas in Sexual Reorientation Therapy　　87
A. Lee Beckstead, PhD

Therapeutic Antidotes: Helping Gay and Bisexual Men
　Recover from Conversion Therapies　　117
Douglas C. Haldeman, PhD

Ethical Issues in Sexual Orientation Conversion Therapies:
　An Empirical Study of Consumers　　131
Michael Schroeder, PsyD
Ariel Shidlo, PhD

Overview of Ethical and Research Issues in Sexual Orientation
    Therapy   167
      Marshall Forstein, MD

Ethical Concerns Raised When Patients Seek to Change
    Same-Sex Attractions   181
      Jack Drescher, MD

Index   211

ABOUT THE EDITORS

Ariel Shidlo, PhD, is a psychologist at the Columbia Center for Gay, Lesbian, and Bisexual Mental Health of Columbia/Presbyterian Medical Center and is also in private practice in New York City. Dr. Shidlo received his PhD in clinical/community psychology from the State University of New York at Buffalo. His research is in the areas of internalized homophobia, HIV-related high-risk sexual behavior, and sexual orientation conversion therapies.

Michael Schroeder, PsyD, is a psychologist in private practice in New York City. He is a former faculty member of the Albert Einstein College of Medicine and received his PsyD in clinical psychology from the Minnesota School of Professional Psychology. Dr. Schroeder's research interests include human sexuality, ethics, and sexual orientation conversion therapies.

Jack Drescher, MD, Editor-in-Chief of the Journal of Gay and Lesbian Psychotherapy, is Supervisor of Psychoanalysis and Faculty Member at the William Alanson White Psychoanalytic Institute and Clinical Assistant Professor of Psychiatry at the State University of New York at Brooklyn. Dr. Drescher chairs both the Committee on Gay, Lesbian and Bisexual Issues of the American Psychiatric Association and the Committee on Human Sexuality of the Group for the Advancement of Psychiatry. Author of *Psychoanalytic Therapy and the Gay Man* (1998, The Analytic Press), Dr. Drescher is in full-time private practice in New York City.

What Needs Fixing?
An Introduction

The American Psychiatric Association's 1973 decision to remove homosexuality as a mental disorder from the *Diagnostic and Statistical Manual of Mental Disorders* (Bayer, 1981) has been followed by an era of significant improvements in the sociopolitical standing of lesbians, gay men, and bisexuals in the United States. Despite these changes, and perhaps even because of them, a marginal subset of mental health practitioners continues to diagnose and treat individuals with a homosexual orientation as if they were mentally ill. The tools these clinicians have used include–either exclusively or sometimes in combination–psychoanalysis, religious faith healing, aversive behavioral conditioning and even electroshock therapy.

While none of these approaches has successfully produced heterosexuality in the majority of patients treated, the practitioners of sexual conversion therapies regard any chance of heterosexual conversion as being worth the effort. Disturbingly, in their therapeutic fervor–if not ideological or religious zeal–to create heterosexuals, reparative or sexual conversion therapists tend to overlook and dismiss any possible harmful side effects of such treatments. In their efforts to save (or recruit?) any potential heterosexual they may encounter, these therapists have appeared almost universally indifferent about inflicting damage upon the self-esteem of those patients who do not become heterosexual and who eventually go on to adopt gay or lesbian identities. In other words, these therapists, and often the larger heterosexual society as well, seem not to care how many gay people are hurt in the process of producing a few more heterosexuals. To counterbalance these serious clinical and ethical omissions, this special issue of the *Journal of Gay & Lesbian Psychotherapy* presents current perspectives, both from patients and clinicians, on the harmful impact of sex-

[Haworth co-indexing entry note]: "What Needs Fixing? An Introduction." Shidlo, Ariel, Michael Schroeder, and Jack Drescher. Co-published simultaneously in *Journal of Gay & Lesbian Psychotherapy* (The Haworth Medical Press, an imprint of The Haworth Press, Inc.) Vol. 5, No. 3/4, 2001, pp. 1-4; and: *Sexual Conversion Therapy: Ethical, Clinical and Research Perspectives* (ed: Ariel Shidlo, Michael Schroeder, and Jack Drescher) The Haworth Medical Press, an imprint of The Haworth Press, Inc., 2001, pp. 1-4. Single or multiple copies of this article are available for a fee from The Haworth Document Delivery Service [1-800-HAWORTH, 9:00 a.m. - 5:00 p.m. (EST). E-mail address: getinfo@haworthpressinc.com].

1

ual orientation conversion interventions. It is the first time that such a wide range of papers on this issue have been gathered together in one volume.

Much of the writing on conversion therapy has been clinician-centered, ignoring, to varying degrees, the wider scope of meanings, emotions and experiences of the individuals who undertake these interventions. Furthermore, in recent years the conversion therapy movement has adopted an infomercial approach–in full-page ads in major American newspapers–which trumpet their successes and attack those who criticize their failures. However, we believe that to better understand the fuller psychological and social dimensions of conversion therapies, it is necessary to give voice to the range of individuals who have sought them out. This allows the accumulation of social scientific data to go beyond reductionist questions of efficacy and outcome and to shed light on what exactly is involved in undertaking the process of fighting against one's homosexual orientation. As a case in point, in contrast to many overly-optimistic and simplified papers by practitioners of conversion therapies, our volume presents Beckstead's report on self-perceived successes by reparative therapy patients. In it, he offers a more in-depth view of the complexity of subjective perceptions of such treatments.

One goal in putting this volume together is to illustrate the sociocultural matrix in which individuals engage professionals (and faith healers) to try to eradicate their desire for sexual and emotional intimacy with persons of the same sex. Toward that end, this volume includes first-hand accounts of persons who have gone through conversion therapies. Two of these essays are written by psychotherapists who underwent these treatments themselves. In addition to conceptual examinations of the history and ethics of conversion therapies, we present empirical data on the ethics of actual current clinical practices of conversion therapists. Finally, we present ideas on processes that can be used to help survivors recover from failed conversion therapies.

"I'm Your Handyman: A History of Reparative Therapies," represents Jack Drescher's 1998 article, first published in the *Journal of Homosexuality*. "Handyman" reviews the history and theoretical assumptions of psychoanalytically-oriented practitioners, beginning with Freud's juvenilization of gay people to the later analysts who pathologized and attempted to change same-sex attractions. Drescher documents the evolution of some reparative therapists from mental health concerned practitioners into antigay political activists. In the process, he provides a powerful illustration of the sometimes permeable boundaries between clinical and political issues.

Paul Moor's "The View from Irving Bieber's Couch: 'Heads I Win, Tails You Lose,'" written for this volume, gives an account of a painful journey into and out of psychoanalysis with one of the leading public figures in the conversion therapy movement of the twentieth century: the late Irving Bieber (Bieber et al., 1962). Moor, who now lives as a music critic in Berlin, writes articulately on the impossible transference demands and subsequent hurtfulness of a therapy motivated by a therapist's agenda to change a patient's sexual orientation.

The volume then goes on to feature some excerpts from Martin Duberman's *Cures: A Gay Man's Odyssey.* In his autobiographical account of trying to be "cured" of his homosexuality, Duberman poignantly reveals the frame of mind of those seeking conversion therapy. He articulates the cognitive manipulations and self-deceit that a conversion candidate must exercise–a mental gymnasium in which the gymnast can find no rest. In his account of his many therapies–including a loss of time and energy and the experience of psychological manipulation by clinicians–Duberman provides a vivid, albeit painful glimpse into why such therapies failed him.

In "Becoming Gay: A Personal Odyssey," openly gay psychoanalyst Richard Isay documents his own efforts to change his homosexual orientation. In this reprinting of a chapter from his 1996 book, *Becoming Gay,* Isay provides a highly personalized account of his initial recognition that he was "homosexual," of his entrance into a heterosexual marriage, and of his struggles to come to term with his gay identity. Isay's journey through a ten-year psychoanalysis demonstrates a common phenomenon: gay identity development placed in stasis, since failed conversion therapies often consume many years in the progression toward development of a gay identity.

"Healing Homosexuals: A Psychologist's Journey Through the Ex-Gay Movement and the Pseudo-Science of Reparative Therapy" is by psychotherapist and former ex-gay leader Jeff Ford. He provides a gripping account of his journey, from youth through adulthood, as a gay man struggling to become straight. He provides the former insider's detailed understanding of the complexities of the ex-gay movement: of its theology, and the ways in which unhappy gay men and lesbians find their way into those organizations. Ford's own attempts to change included entering into a heterosexual marriage, adopting a child, electroshock therapy, psychotherapy, attending Homosexuals Anonymous, and a total immersion–which included a leadership position–in ex-gay ministries.

A. Lee Beckstead's "Cures versus Choices: Agendas in Sexual Reorientation Therapy" examines the perspectives of 20 religious clients of conversion therapies. He draws upon these data to develop a conceptual framework for understanding the heterogeneity of meanings in those individuals whose positive experiences with conversion therapies stem from a commitment to antihomosexual religious beliefs which overrides any commitment to taking on a gay or lesbian sexual identity.

Douglas C. Haldeman's "Therapeutic Antidotes: Helping Gay and Bisexual Men Recover from Conversion Therapies" describes the author's twenty years of clinical experiences with post-conversion therapy "refugees." In his work with these patients, he focuses on the areas of depression related to loss, intimacy avoidance, sexual dysfunction, demasculinization and spirituality, and religion. His use of case examples provides a clinical context for understanding and helping patients who are recovering from unsuccessful conversion therapies.

In "Ethical Issues in Sexual Orientation Conversion Therapies: An Empirical Study of Consumers," Michael Schroeder and Ariel Shidlo provide documentation, based on patient reports, of poor and questionable clinical practice as well as ethical violations by licensed mental health practitioners. Based on their 150 interviews with conversion therapy consumers, this seminal study is the first to provide significant empirical data demonstrating how conversion therapies can violate professional codes of conduct regarding informed consent, confidentiality, pre-termination counseling and provision of referrals after treatment failure.

In "Overview of Ethical and Research Issues in Sexual Orientation Therapy," Marshall Forstein presents an analysis of the conceptual challenges involved in conducting meaningful research on sexual orientation conversion therapies. He also examines inherent ethical difficulties in the application of conversion therapies and proposes some guidelines to remedy them. Finally, Forstein illuminates the inter-connectedness of political power, social control, religion, morality, medicine, and psychotherapy, and the impact of values and bias on science and clinical practice.

Jack Drescher's "Ethical Concerns Raised When Patients Seek to Change Same-Sex Attractions" was written expressly for this volume. In it, he advances the arguments of his previous paper to counter the specious claim–made by conversion therapists–that therapists have an ethical responsibility to refer individuals with antihomosexual religious beliefs to reparative therapists in order to change their sexual identities. He places this argument in the context of the culture wars surrounding homosexuality and notes that the reported experiences of former patients should give reasonable pause to clinicians before referring anyone to a reparative therapist.

Ariel Shidlo, PhD
Michael Schroeder, PsyD
Jack Drescher, MD

REFERENCES

Bayer, R. (1981), *Homosexuality and American Psychiatry: The Politics of Diagnosis.* New York: Basic Books.

Bieber, I., Dain, H., Dince, P., Drellich, M., Grand, H., Gundlach, R., Kremer, M., Rifkin, A., Wilbur, C., & Bieber T. (1962), *Homosexuality: A Psychoanalytic Study.* New York: Basic Books.

Duberman, M. (1991), *Cures: A Gay Man's Odyssey.* New York: Dutton.

Isay, R. (1996), *Becoming Gay: The Journey to Self-Acceptance.* New York: Pantheon.

I'm Your Handyman:
A History of Reparative Therapies

Jack Drescher, MD

SUMMARY. Reparative therapy has come to generically define talking cures that claim to change an individual's homosexual orientation to a heterosexual one. Although other treatment modalities have also promised to "cure" homosexuality, the history of reparative therapies has become inexorably linked with that of psychoanalysis. This paper reviews the history and theoretical assumptions of psychoanalytically-oriented practitioners, beginning with Freud's juvenilization of gay people to the later analysts who pathologized and attempted to change same-sex attractions. The evolution of reparative therapists from medically concerned practitioners into antigay political activists is also discussed. The evolution of one branch of psychoanalytic theory into an antihomosexual political movement illustrates the permeability of boundaries between clinical issues and political ones. In their open support of antigay legislation, reparative therapists have moved from the traditional psychoanalytic center and have been embraced by conservative religious and political forces opposed to homosexuality. In doing so, they have appar-

Jack Drescher is Training and Supervising Analyst at the William Alanson White Psychoanalytic Institute; Editor-in-Chief of the *Journal of Gay & Lesbian Psychotherapy* and author of *Psychoanalytic Therapy and the Gay Man* (The Analytic Press); Immediate Past President of the New York County District Branch of the APA and a member of its Committee on Ethics. Dr. Drescher is in private practice in New York City.

Address correspondence to: Jack Drescher, 420 West 23rd Street, #7D, New York, NY 10011 (E-mail: jadres@psychoanalysis.net).

This article was originally published in the *Journal of Homosexuality*, Volume 36, Number 1, 1998. © 1998 by The Haworth Press, Inc. All rights reserved.

[Haworth co-indexing entry note]: "I'm Your Handyman: A History of Reparative Therapies." Drescher, Jack. Co-published simultaneously in *Journal of Gay & Lesbian Psychotherapy* (The Haworth Medical Press, an imprint of The Haworth Press, Inc.) Vol. 5, No. 3/4, 2001, pp. 5-24; and: *Sexual Conversion Therapy: Ethical, Clinical and Research Perspectives* (ed: Ariel Shidlo, Michael Schroeder, and Jack Drescher) The Haworth Medical Press, an imprint of The Haworth Press, Inc., 2001, pp. 5-24. Single or multiple copies of this article are available for a fee from The Haworth Document Delivery Service [1-800-HAWORTH, 9:00 a.m. - 5:00 p.m. (EST). E-mail address: getinfo@haworthpressinc.com].

ently adopted religious organizational practices themselves, preaching dogma and stifling dissent. The increasing marginalization of reparative therapists from the psychoanalytic mainstream illustrates how psychoanalysis *per se* is neither gay-affirming nor condemning, although psychoanalytic practitioners may fall into either of these categories. *[Article copies available for a fee from The Haworth Document Delivery Service: 1-800-HAWORTH. E-mail address: <getinfo@haworthpressinc.com> Website: <http://www.HaworthPress.com>]*

KEYWORDS. Antihomosexual bias, bisexuality, developmental theory, Freud, gay and lesbian patients, homosexuality, psychiatric ethics, psychotherapy, psychoanalysis, reparative therapy, respect for patients, sexual conversion therapy

INTRODUCTION

Homosexuality is assuredly no advantage, but it is nothing to be ashamed of, no vice, no degradation; it cannot be classified as an illness; we consider it to be a variation of the sexual function, produced by a certain arrest of sexual development . . .

–Sigmund Freud
Letter to an American Mother (1935)

Although psychoanalysts have proffered and claimed homosexual conversions since the time of Freud, a recently coined term, *reparative therapy* (Nicolosi, 1991), has come to generically define talking cures that claim to change an individual's homosexual orientation to a heterosexual one. Although other treatment modalities such as aversion therapies and psychosurgery have also promised to "cure" homosexuality, the history of reparative therapies has become inexorably linked with that of psychoanalysis. The strident positions of reparative theorists and practitioners (Bayer, 1981; Socarides, 1994b; Socarides et al., 1997; Drescher, 1997, 1998a), and the tacit acquiescence of their less ideological colleagues, have earned psychoanalytic theory its present mythic status as an implacable foe of lesbian and gay identities. This view persists despite a growing number of authors who criticize the antihomosexual bias of psychoanalytic theories within a psychoanalytic framework (Morgenthaler, 1988; Friedman, 1988; Lewes, 1988; Isay, 1989; O'Connor & Ryan, 1993; Glassgold & Iasenza, 1995; Domenici & Lesser, 1995; D'Ercole, 1996; Kiersky, 1996). The perception that psychoanalysis is intrinsically hostile to homosexuality led the reviewer of a book affirmatively reformulating psychoanalytic theory and practice with lesbians and gay men (Domenici & Lesser, 1995) to skeptically muse: "Some of the contributors discuss how they are readapting or selectively using psychoanalysis so that its inherent antigay bias is eliminated. If that bias is eliminated, what is left?" (Marrow, 1996).

This paper reviews the history and theoretical assumptions of psychoanalytically-oriented practitioners, beginning with Freud's juvenilization of gay people to the later analysts who pathologized and attempted to change same-sex attractions. The evolution of reparative therapists from medically concerned practitioners into antigay political activists is also discussed.

FREUD

It is not for psycho-analysis to solve the problem of homosexuality.

–Sigmund Freud
Psychogenesis of a Case of Homosexuality in a Woman (1920)

Although he never dedicated a major work solely to the subject of homosexuality, Freud's contributions on the subject range across a period of almost twenty years (1905, 1908, 1909, 1910, 1911, 1914, 1920, 1923). The contradictions in his voluminous works make Freud's position opaque to the casual, modern reader. Attempts to find "the real Freud" are too often motivated by those who seek his agreement with their own point of view. When diametrically opposed camps claim Freud as a theoretical ally, it confirms Bayer's (1981) assertion that "The status of homosexuality is a political question, representing a historically rooted, socially determined choice regarding the ends of human sexuality" (p. 5). Taken out of the historical context in which he wrote, and depending upon the author's selective citations, Freud can be portrayed as either virulently antihomosexual (Nicolosi, 1991) or as a closeted friend of gays (McWilliams, 1996). This section is an attempt to offer a portrait of Freud's complex position in the historical context in which he theorized and lived.

Freud's attitude toward homosexuality was tolerant for its time. He signed a statement calling for decriminalization of homosexual acts in 1930s Germany and Austria (Abelove, 1986). This action was based on his belief that people should not be treated as criminals if their behaviors originated from a "psychic disposition" beyond their control. Unlike today's reparative therapists, Freud did not believe that criminalization and social opprobrium were acceptable therapeutic tools. He also empathically noted, "It is one of the obvious social injustices that the standard of civilization should demand from everyone the same conduct of sexual life–conduct which can be followed without any difficulty by some people, thanks to their organization, but which imposes the heaviest psychical sacrifices on others" (Freud, 1908, p. 192). In disputing degeneracy theory's (Krafft-Ebing, 1886) pejorative views, Freud observed that homosexuality is " . . . found in people whose efficiency is unimpaired, and who are indeed distinguished by specially high intellectual development and ethical culture" (Freud, 1905, p. 138).

Freud believed a sublimated homosexuality was necessary for normal heterosexual function. Similarly, all homosexuals had some heterosexual feelings. There was no social equivalent of "coming out" in Freud's era and so he never expressed an opinion on that subject. However, one can surmise he did not believe overt homosexual behavior was socially acceptable. Freud scolds a patient who asks why people shouldn't express their homosexual feelings as well as their heterosexual ones:

> Normal people have a certain homosexual component and a very strong heterosexual component. The homosexual component should be sublimated as it now is in society; it is one of the most valuable human assets, and should be put to social uses. One cannot give one's impulses free rein. Your attitude reminds me of a child who just discovered everybody defecates and who then demands that everybody ought to defecate in public; that cannot be. (Wortis, 1954, pp. 99-100)

A significant difficulty in understanding Freud's work stems from the fact that when discussing homosexuality, he is primarily elaborating other theoretical concepts such as libido and bisexuality (1905), narcissism (1910, 1914), projective mechanisms (1911, 1923), or unsatisfactory Oedipal resolutions (1920, 1923). Because each is addressing a different metapsychological issue, Freud's four theories of homosexuality (Lewes, 1988) are often contradictory. Each uses a narrowly constructed *hypothetical homosexual* (Drescher, 1998b) to make a different theoretical point.

Moreover, Freud's position on homosexuality cannot be understood in the language of the contemporary debate about homosexuality. In fact, his *original intent* is sometimes obscured when his opinions are brought into the modern controversy. For example, in a posthumously published *Letter to an American Mother* (1935), Freud reassured a woman that her homosexual son was not ill. In the late 20th century it is argued that lesbians and gay men are not ill and their homosexuality is defined as intrinsic to their nature (LeVay, 1993; Hamer & Copeland, 1994). It follows, according to this argument, that lesbians and gay men should be accorded minority status and full civil rights.

Although similar arguments were made by Magnus Hirschfeld (Bullough, 1979) in Freud's time, they were not germane to his letter. Freud was using the term *illness* as a synonym for symptom formation, by which he meant the product of intrapsychic conflict (1926). Homosexuality was not defined as an illness because it was thought to represent the unconflicted expression of an infantile sexual wish (Freud, 1905; 1920). However, although an arrested libidinal development was not an illness, neither did Freud believe that it implied health (Drescher, 1996b). In Freud's view, one could still justify psychotherapeutic intervention to transform a person's sexual orientation.

Freud theorized that early childhood development was organized into psychosexual stages of libido. This hierarchical ordering of pleasure moved from oral to anal to genital stages. It placed genital (heterosexual) intercourse above the former, more infantile forms of gratification. Adult sexuality was defined as genital-genital (penile-vaginal) intercourse and oral and anal sexuality were labeled as foreplay or immature vestiges of childhood sexual expression. Homosexuality could be due to a *libidinal arrest* or failure to reach the final psychosexual stage of genitality due to a blockage of the energic force. An alternative explanation was that an individual had reached the more mature, genital stage but due to trauma reverted to an earlier stage. This was termed a *libidinal regression*. For Freud, changing an individual's same-sex orientation to a heterosexual one meant helping them achieve a higher level of psychosexual development. Rather than a cure, effecting a sexual orientation conversion was seen as a metaphor for helping the patient grow up. Thus, in qualifying his reassurances to the "American Mother," Freud explained that illness was not a necessary criterion for change:

> By asking me if I can help, you mean, I suppose, if I can abolish homosexuality and make normal heterosexuality take its place. The answer is, in a general way, we cannot promise to achieve it. In a certain number of cases we succeed in developing the blighted germs of heterosexual tendencies which are present in every homosexual, in the majority of cases it is no more possible. (Freud, 1935)

In *Psychogenesis of a Case of Homosexuality in a Woman* (1920), Freud documents a reparative therapy attempt. This is his only reported case in which he is nominally charged with changing someone's sexual orientation. His patient was an eighteen-year-old girl who had fallen in love with an older woman. Following a stern rebuke from her father, the young woman attempted suicide. She was subsequently brought by her parents for psychoanalytic treatment to change her sexual orientation. In the paper, Freud pointed out the difficulties in achieving the father's goal for his teenage daughter:

> . . . parents expect one to cure their nervous and unruly child. By a healthy child they mean one who never causes his parents trouble, and gives them nothing but pleasure. The physician may succeed in curing

the child, but after that it goes its own way all the more decidedly, and the parents are now far more dissatisfied than before. In short, it is not a matter of indifference whether someone comes to analysis of his own accord or because he is brought to it–whether it is he himself who desires to be changed, or only his relatives, who love him (or who might be expected to love him). Further unfavorable features in the present case were the facts that the girl was not in any way ill (she did not suffer from anything in herself, nor did she complain of her condition) and that the task to be carried out did not consist in resolving a neurotic conflict but in converting one variety of the genital organization of sexuality into the other. Such an achievement–the removal of genital inversion or homosexuality–is in my experience never an easy matter. . . . In general, to undertake to convert a fully developed homosexual into a heterosexual does not offer much prospect of success than the reverse, except that for good practical reasons the latter is never attempted. (p. 150)

Freud hypothesized that the young woman's early oedipal rivalry with her mother was reactivated in puberty when her parents had another child:

It was just when the girl was experiencing the revival of her infantile Oedipus complex at puberty that she suffered her great disappointment. She became keenly conscious of the wish to have a child, and a male one; that what she desired was her *father's* child and an image of *him*, her consciousness was not allowed to know. And what happened next? It was not *she* who bore the child, but her unconsciously hated rival, her mother. Furiously resentful and embittered, she turned away from her father and from men altogether. After this first great reverse she forswore her womanhood and sought another goal for her libido. (p. 157)

Freud called his lesbian patient a spurned man-hater, labeled her dreams as "false and hypocritical" (p. 165), and disparaged her as a feminist who suffered from penis envy (p. 169). He claimed *her* transferential animosity toward men was an insurmountable obstacle that forced him to end the treatment and exile her lesbian desire (Kiersky, 1996). He advised the family to have the young woman continue with a female analyst. No report of the existence, success or failure of any subsequent treatment is known. However that report was irrelevant to Freud's purposes, because the aim of this paper was to further expand upon his previous psychoanalytic theories. In fact, the unsatisfactory outcome of the case only confirmed the correctness of Freud's views that homosexuality was not a neurosis, but a difficult-to-treat psychic disposition.

REPARATIVE THERAPY'S GILDED AGE

The psychiatrists were always in desperate need to find a biological foundation for homosexuality; in their fight against barbaric, medieval laws, naturally they picked upon inherited homosexuality.

–Sandor Rado (Roazen & Swerdloff, 1995)

Despite Freud's pessimism about changing homosexual motivations to heterosexual ones, analysts persisted in seeking ways to do so. Psychoanalysts were in the vanguard of redefining socially denigrated behaviors in psychological terms and consequently generated the hope that medical intervention might be able to change them. When psychoanalysis reached its highest influence in psychiatry and academia during the 1940s and through the 1960s, many gay men and women voluntarily sought psychoanalytic treatment for their same-sex feelings (Duberman, 1991; Isay, 1996).

Although Freud's libidinal model offered little hope for converting homosexuality, psychoanalytic opinion began to change. After Freud's death in 1938 (Jones, 1961), psychoanalytic theories proliferated that differed significantly from his own but that nevertheless remained within the mainstream of the psychoanalytic movement (Greenberg & Mitchell, 1983). These new paradigms offered alternative explanations for same-sex attraction that created "therapeutic possibilities." In the post-Freudian psychoanalytic world, the theories of Sandor Rado laid the foundations for what would later come to be called "reparative therapies."

RADO

Rado's (1969)[1] theory of homosexuality grew out of the refutation of Freud's belief in psychological bisexuality. Rado believed the theory of libidinal bisexuality was based on a faulty analogy with anatomical bisexuality. That is, underlying Freud's theory was the later-disproved 19th-century belief in embryonic hermaphroditism, the hypothesis that the potential to become an anatomical man or a woman was present in every embryo (Rado, 1969, pp. 215-216). However, after Rado deconstructed Freud's biological metaphors, he succumbed to the same epistemological snare. He too relied upon the physiological and evolutionary models *of his own era* as concrete metaphors for psychological experience:

In *adaptational psychodynamics* we analyze behavior in the context of a biological organism interacting with its cultural environment. The human organism, like other living organisms, may be defined as a self-regulating biological system that perpetuates itself and its type by means of its environment, its surrounding system. From this it follows that life is a process of interaction of the organism and its environment. . . . In the theory of evolution, the crowning achievement of eighteenth and nineteen-century biologists, *adaptive value is a statistical concept which epitomizes reproductive efficiency* in a certain environment. This is strongly influenced by the type's ability to survive. Hence, "more adaptive" means more able to survive and reproduce. (1969, p. 4, emphasis added)

Rado declared, with great authority but without any supporting scientific research or evidence, that heterosexuality is the only nonpathological outcome of human sexual development: "I know of nothing that indicates that there is any such thing as innate orgastic desire for a partner of the same sex" (1969, p. 210). Starting from that unproven, but firmly-held assumption, he offered the following theory of homosexuality's etiology:

The male-female sexual pattern is dictated by anatomy . . . by means of the institution of marriage, the male-female sexual pattern is culturally ingrained and perpetuated in every individual from earliest childhood . . . [homosexual] pairs satisfy their repudiated yet irresistible male-female desire by means of shared illusions and actual approximations; such is the hold on the individual of a cultural institution based on biological foundations. . . . Why is the so-called homosexual forced to escape from the male-female pair into a homogenous pair? . . . the familiar campaign of deterrence that parents wage to prohibit the sexual activity of the child. The campaign causes the female to view the male organ as a destructive weapon. Therefore the female partners are reassured by the absence in both of them of the male organ. The campaign causes the male to see in the mutilated female organ a reminder of inescapable punishment. When . . . fear and resentment of the opposite organ becomes insurmountable, the individual may escape into homosexuality. The male patterns are reassured by the presence in both of them of the male organ. Homosexuality is a deficient adaptation evolved by the organism in response to its own emergency overreaction and dyscontrol. (pp. 212-213)

BIEBER

Bieber, Dain et al. (1962) conducted a psychoanalytic study that they claimed confirmed Rado's theory of homosexuality: constitutional factors were insignificant and parental psychopathology was the cause of homosexuality. They examined 106 homosexual men and 100 male heterosexual controls in psychoanalytic treatment to identify family patterns presumed to be responsible for homosexuality. The authors' initial assumptions were consistent with the theory they subsequently claimed to confirm: "We have selected the patient-mother-father unit for analysis. . . . We believe that personality for the most part is forged within the triangular system of the nuclear family. It follows then that personality maladaptation must also be primarily rooted here" (pp. 140-141). "We assume that heterosexuality is the biologic norm and that unless interfered with all individuals are heterosexual" (p. 319). "We consider homosexuality to be a pathologic biosocial, psychosexual adaptation consequent to pervasive fears surrounding the expression of heterosexual impulses. In our view, every homosexual is, in reality, a 'latent' heterosexual" (p. 220). They claimed that of their 106 homosexual men, "29 patients had become exclusively heterosexual during the course of psychoanalytic treatment. The shift from homosexuality to exclusive heterosexuality for 27 per cent of the H[omosexual]-patients is of outstanding importance since these are the most optimistic and promising results thus far reported" (p. 276).

SOCARIDES I

Socarides contests Freud's view that homosexuality is a developmental arrest and redefines it as conflictual. His conflict model suggests therapeutic interventions to bring unconscious struggles into awareness in order to reduce homosexual symptoms. He reshapes Freud's (1926) metapsychological constructs and claims that homosexuality is a neurotic condition in which the libidinal instinct has "undergone excessive transformation and disguise in order to be gratified in the perverse act. The perverted action, like the neurotic symptom, results from the conflict between the ego and the id and represents a compromise formation which at the same time must be acceptable to the demands of the superego . . . the instinctual gratification takes place in disguised form while its real content remains unconscious" (Socarides, 1968, pp. 35-36). Because homosexuality is now defined as a compromise between intrapsychic forces, it meets the psychoanalytic definition of an illness. His claims, like Freud's, are neither provable or unprovable since the metapsychological constructs of id, ego and superego are not subject to direct observation and can only be understood inferentially.

Socarides holds the parents of gay men and women responsible for causing homosexuality. The recent emergence of his gay son from the closet (Nagourney, 1995; Dunlap, 1995) adds poignancy to his 30-year-old description of the fathers of homosexual men: "The family of the homosexual is usually a female-dominated environment wherein the father was absent, weak, detached or sadistic" (Socarides, 1968, p. 38). Socarides also claims a psychoanalytic conversion rate of 35% for his homosexual patients (1995, p. 102).

OVESEY

Ovesey's (1969) work approaches the post-modern sensibility in his explanation of how categories of masculinity and femininity are socially constructed:

> The social order is so arranged that status accrues to men solely by virtue of the fact that they are men. The polarities of masculinity and femininity are identified respectively with positive and negative value judgments. Masculinity represents strength, dominance, superiority; femininity represents weakness, submissiveness, inferiority. The former is equated with success; the latter with failure. It is true that these values are cultural stereotypes that express primarily the historical prejudices of the men in the culture. However, it would be safe to say that men and women alike make use of them in appraising each other's behavior. (p. 76)

Men who have dreams or fantasies in which they appear submissive to or dependent upon other men are not necessarily experiencing homosexual feelings, but *pseudohomosexual* ones. These feelings are symbolic of competition and status issues commonly found in heterosexual men. Despite his awareness of how cultural forces value masculine attributes while feminine ones are denigrated, Ovesey treats male homosexuality's low cultural status as a fact of nature that requires no further deconstruction. In fact, he warned that "those who lack conviction that homosexuality is a treatable illness, but believe instead that it is a natural constitutional variant, should not accept homosexuals as patients" (p. 119).

In Ovesey's approach to treating male homosexuality, we see the standard recommendation of reparative therapists to abandon neutrality or objectivity and function as behavioral therapists: "There is only one way that the homosexual can overcome this phobia and learn to have heterosexual intercourse, and that way is in bed with a woman. . . . Sooner or later, the homosexual patient must make the necessary attempts to have intercourse, and he must make them again and again, until he is capable of a sustained erection, penetration, and pleasurable intravaginal orgasm" (pp. 106-107). In order to achieve these goals, the reparative therapist becomes a dating consultant for the patient:

> Most homosexuals do not move readily toward women. More often, the patient protests that he is not ready for sex with a woman. He is, of course, right. The therapist should reassure him that for the present he is

only asked to see women socially, to date them; nobody is asking that he jump into bed with them. Later, when he is comfortable with a date, he will begin first to neck, then to pet, and eventually go even further, but certainly not now. If the patient is at all serious about treatment, he will accept this compromise and gradually, with some pressure from the therapist, if necessary, begin to go out. . . . There is a place, just as in the therapy of other phobias, where the patient may be threatened with termination if he unduly procrastinates about entering the phobic situation. In other words, the homosexual patient should be given an ultimatum for insufficient efforts to perform heterosexually. . . . (pp. 120-121)

CONTEMPORARY REPARATIVE THERAPY: TRADITIONAL VALUES FOR A POSTMODERN ERA

We refused most emphatically to turn a patient who puts himself into our hands in search of help into our private property, to decide his fate for him, to force our own ideals upon him, and with the pride of a Creator to form him in our own image and see that it is good . . . we cannot accept (the) proposal either–namely that psycho-analysis should place itself in the service of a particular philosophical outlook on the world and should urge this upon the patient for the purpose of ennobling his mind. In my opinion, this is after all only to use violence, even though it is overlaid with the most honorable motives.

–Sigmund Freud
Lines of Advance in Psycho-Analytic Therapy (1918)

Rado's adaptational model of homosexuality dominated American psychiatry until a year after his death in 1972 (Roazen & Swerdloff, 1995). In 1973, the American Psychiatric Association deleted homosexuality from its *Diagnostic and Statistical Manual* (Bayer, 1981). Although Rado's theory is no longer the dominant mental health paradigm, it continues to surface in new forms.

Contemporary reparative therapists must contend with the fact that the terms of scientific and social debate have shifted. They have had to grapple with five significant factors that their predecessors did not: (1) Their patients and potential patients are aware of affirmative identities for lesbians and gay men as that community's public visibility increases; (2) there is a growing, significant scientific and social science literature that defines homosexuality as a normal variant of human sexuality; (3) rigid categories of masculinity and femininity are being increasingly deconstructed by feminist and queer theorists; (4) there is a growing body of research on antihomosexual attitudes; and (5) homosexuality's diagnostic status as an illness has been rejected by conservative psychoanalytic organizations.[2] Despite these cultural changes, the theoretical formulations underlying reparative therapies have changed little since the time of Rado. However, as the following section illustrates, reparative therapists have modified their rhetorical strategies in their adherence to traditional approaches to homosexuality. They have also moved beyond rhetoric to significant political action.

SIEGEL: THE NEOCON

In the reparative therapy literature, Siegel (1988) prefaces her work by presenting herself as an accidental tourist, for whom "a series of coincidences placed me into the position of analyzing twelve women who thought they had 'chosen' homosexuality as a lifestyle" (p. xi). She identifies herself as a reparative therapy neoconservative, a former liberal whose clinical experiences have led her to regard her previous, more tolerant beliefs as part of an idealistic youth that she has disavowed for a new, albeit unpopular, truth:

> My [lesbian] patients had convinced me on an irrational level that there was indeed a choice for them . . . To be a liberal and liberated woman and yet to review homosexuality as the result of untoward development seemed at times a betrayal of all I then believed. But viewing my patients through the lens of psychoanalytic thinkers and clinicians soon showed me that allowing myself to be seduced into perceiving female homosexuality as a normal lifestyle would have cemented both my patients and myself into a rigid mode that precluded change of whatever nature. (p. xii)

In her treatment of twelve lesbian patients, Siegel claims more than half became "fully heterosexual." She defines homosexuality as preoedipal in origin. In the Radoite tradition, she believes her patients "tried to heal their defective body images by seeking others like themselves" (p. 8). She bases her work on the theories of Socarides (1968, 1978), to whom she dedicates her book. Like Socarides, she uses Mahler's (et al., 1975) model of separation and individuation as universal metaphors of normal development.

As reparative therapy increasingly moves away from the scientific mainstream, its mystical presuppositions become more apparent. Siegel, for example, defines the psychoanalytic concept of narcissism as "an energy" which allows individuals to adapt to "the reality of life, what I have called *Lebensbejahung*, the cathexis of life" (p. 21). In the tradition of classical psychoanalysis, she interprets from what she believes to be an objective position and has an inflated sense of her own capacity for neutrality. She presents her clinical narratives as historical facts that she has unearthed in the course of analysis. Her approach is somewhat formulaic, marked by a belief that all her patients go through similar "stages" of transference phenomena. She would have her readers believe she had no preconceived ideas about homosexuality or heterosexuality and came to her eventual conclusion that homosexuality is pathological through a scientific process of observation. It is beyond the scope of this paper to address the influence of the analyst's beliefs on the narratives that emerge in a patient's treatment and the subject has been addressed elsewhere (Drescher, 1996a). However, Siegel's clinical approach appears to undermine her own attempts to position her work among self-psychology and intersubjective theorists, given their emphasis on co-constructed narratives.

NICOLOSI: THE MORAL MAJORITY[3]

Psychoanalytic theorists traditionally couched their moral condemnations of homosexuality within scientific and pseudo-scientific metaphors. The Radoite tradition, in particular, anthropomorphized the concept of evolution, turning it into a force of nature that "expected" individuals to behave in ways for which they were designed. Consequently, the will of the deity was replaced by the will of evolution in psychoanalytic literature. This approach is embodied in the work of Kardiner:

> . . . sex morality is not an arbitrary set of rules set down by no one knows who, and for purposes that no one understands, but is what man found expedient in his long evolutionary march, his social evolution. . . . If we find a culture, such as our own, that not only has survived but has to its credit the highest accomplishments ever recorded for man, then the patterns of morality–or the mores by which it governs the relations of the constituents to one another–must have a high degree of effectiveness . . . at the time sex custom entered recorded history, it already was more or less settled. Monogamy, for example, was an established custom in the Homeric legends . . . we can assume that "human nature" has certain constant features and that human interaction, within certain limits, can be predicted on the basis of man's biological make-up. . . . What is more certain is that in man the capacity for love is more extensive owing to the fact that human infants need the proximity of protecting parents for a longer period than do any other mammals. This dependency is the nucleus about which the emotion known as love develops. (Kardiner, 1955, pp. 22-31)

One can only wonder what Kardiner understood about the relationship between Achilles and Patroclus in *The Iliad*. This moralizing tendency within psychoanalysis did not go unobserved and was subsequently embraced by religious institutions that traditionally condemned psychoanalytic thought. Thus, in a document entitled *The Norms of Priestly Formation,* homosexuality is ironically described in heretical psychoanalytic terminology: "The existence of a close link between emotions and sexuality and their interdependence in the wholeness of a personality cannot be denied, even though these two things are diversely understood. In order to talk about a person as mature, his sexual instinct must have overcome two immature tendencies, narcissism and homosexuality, and must have arrived at heterosexuality" (National Conference of Catholic Bishops, 1982, p. 167).

Nicolosi's (1991) approach marks a significant shift in the reparative therapy literature. This reparative therapist offers a deliberate fusion of spiritual and psychoanalytic thought:

> Each one of us, man and woman alike, is driven by the power of romantic love. These infatuations gain their power from the unconscious drive to become a complete human being. In heterosexuals, it is the drive to bring together the male-female polarity through the longing for the other-than me. But in homosexuals, it is the attempt to fulfill a deficit in wholeness of one's original gender. (pp. 109-110)

In addition to the Radoite theory of homosexuality, Nicolosi draws on literature from the field of pastoral counseling. He offers a religious treatise on homosexuality thinly disguised as a scientific document. In the new religious *cum* scientific paradigm, mental health is defined as conformity to traditional values and norms. Nicolosi's reparative therapy "acknowledges the significance of gender difference, the worth of family and conventional values, and the importance of the prevention of gender confusion in children" (p. 23). He criticizes contemporary normal variant theories of homosexuality with the fervor of a religious fundamentalist. In doing so, he argues not as a scientist, but as a preacher:

> The logic of the following assumption has always eluded me: because perhaps 4 percent of all people are homosexual, then homosexuality *must be a normal variation* of human sexuality. The fact that it occurs in other cultures and in subhuman species, under certain conditions, is also seen to prove its normalcy. Such logic would be equivalent to concluding that since a given percentage of people will break a leg skiing each winter, then a broken leg is a natural condition and one should not attempt to avoid it. (p. 132)

Nicolosi's misuse of psychoanalytic concepts to buttress his moralizing approach has been criticized elsewhere (Drescher, 1998a, b). His entire work is characterized by an idealization of heterosexuality, the use of denigrating stereotypes of gay people, and a tendency to treat his own biases as universal truths:

> Gay couples are characteristically brief and very volatile, with much fighting, arguing, making-up again, and continual disappointments. They may take the form of intense romances, where the attraction remains primarily sexual, characterized by infatuation and never evolving into mature love; or else they settle into long-term friendships while maintaining outside affairs. Research, however, reveals that they almost never possess the mature elements of quiet consistency, trust, mutual dependency, and sexual fidelity characteristic of highly functioning heterosexual marriages. (p. 110)

SOCARIDES II: THE COMEBACK KID

Socarides is the perennial reparative therapist who keeps going and going. He was a prominent opponent of the American Psychiatric Association's decision to delete the diagnosis of homosexuality from its *Diagnostic and Statistical Manual* and a leader in the opposition's clamor for a referendum on the decision. Bayer (1981) remarked, "It [was] rather remarkable that the same psychiatrists who had charged the APA's board with an unscientific and unseemly capitulation to political pressure now invoked the referendum procedure" (p. 142). After losing that political battle, Socarides and other psychoanalysts continued to maintain that homosexuality was always pathological. As a result, while other psychiatric organizations assimilated their lesbian and gay members, psychoanalytic institutions continued to maintain discriminatory policies in training and promotion of lesbian and gay analysts (Drescher, 1995).

In his public announcements, Socarides has amazingly tried to portray himself as a defender of gay rights. In this Orwellian approach, he is referring to an individual's right to seek treatment to change a homosexual orientation: "The homosexual must be granted freedom from persecutory laws as well as full civil rights–and this constitutes an integral part of our approach to homosexual individuals . . . while we ask for civil rights, we also ask for the legitimate psychiatric rights of homosexuals to seek help for what they correctly feel is a disorder" (Socarides, 1994a).

However, despite Socarides' often-repeated opposition to antigay discrimination, he and other reparative therapists filed affidavits *in support* of Colorado's antigay Amendment Two (Socarides, 1993), which was eventually overturned by the Supreme Court. That law would have prevented any municipality from offering civil rights protections specifically to lesbians and gay men. Furthermore, in the case of *Campbell v. Sundquist* (1995), Socarides submitted an affidavit as part of the state's unsuccessful defense of Tennessee's Sodomy laws. His actions are consistent with the reparative therapy belief that social opprobrium must be reinforced if gay men and women are to be motivated to change their homosexual orientations.

In 1991, the American Psychoanalytic Association issued a nondiscriminatory statement regarding the acceptance of lesbian and gay candidates and the promotion of training and supervising analysts in their affiliated institutes (Isay, 1996). This was a *de facto* repudiation of Socarides and his view that homosexuality was always a sign of psychopathology and serious mental illness. However, the rejection of his life's work by the psychoanalytic mainstream did not deter Socarides from seeking out other forums to continue expounding his views. These have included editorials in politically conservative newspapers (Socarides, 1994b; Socarides et al., 1997), a book written for a nonprofessional audience that recycles his pathologizing theories and demonizes his political enemies (Socarides, 1995), and starting an organization of his own with himself as its first President.

NARTH

Diminishing professional interest in their approaches has led reparative therapists to form their own organization: The National Association for Research and Therapy of Homosexuality (NARTH). To avoid any repetition of the embarrassment and defeats they experienced in the clinical, scientific and political debates in other professional organizations, NARTH's officers have taken the position that it is unacceptable for current and potential members to publicly question the group's belief that homosexuality is an illness. To disagree would undermine the organization's *raison d'être* of providing an environment in which reparative therapists do not have their pathologizing beliefs challenged:

> NARTH is an association founded to study homosexuality. We make the assumption that obligatory homosexuality is a treatable disorder. Our members hold many variations of that essential view.
>
> The NARTH officers may opt to deny or remove membership when an individual's written statements or public speeches show a clear antipathy to this position. We do not always choose to exercise this option, but will do so when, in our judgment, a potential member is likely to be disruptive because he or she is blatantly opposed to our goals.
>
> Our criterion of discrimination is philosophical; we do not . . . discriminate on the basis of sexual orientation. In fact, many of our mem-

bers are ex-gays or homosexual people in a state of transition toward heterosexuality. (NARTH, 1996)

Agreement with NARTH'S prevailing dogma appears to be the primary criterion for membership, not an individual's professional background. The heretical belief that homosexuality is a normal variant of human sexuality is unwelcome and those who articulate that view risk excommunication if they voice it publicly. However, neocon converts to NARTH's beliefs, ex-gays and potential ex-gays are always welcome. These organizational approaches are consistent with the activities of a fundamentalist religious denomination, not a scientific association.

In the current political climate, NARTH's dogmatic views have been marginalized in professional and scientific organizations. It is uncertain if NARTH will have some future impact on clinical practice and thought in those mainstream mental health professions that presently accept homosexuality as a normal variant of human sexuality. For the present, however, reparative therapists have demonstrated their willingness to ally themselves with religious denominations that condemn homosexuality. Because they are unable to find reputable scientific support for their positions, these antihomosexual religious organizations have turned to reparative therapists to treat their flocks and to provide a veneer of modern respectability. NARTH, in turn, appears to be emulating the tactics of creationists who obscure their increasingly fundamentalist religious political agendas behind scientific and pseudo-scientific language (Tiffen, 1994). Antihomosexual politics make strange bedfellows and Freud, the devoutest of atheists (Gay, 1987), would find this wedding of psychoanalysis and fundamentalism astonishing.

CONCLUSION

There is no point telling people who have difficulties that they are ill.

–D. W. Winnicott
Talking to Parents (1993)

This paper reviewed the history of psychoanalytic theories of homosexuality and therapies designed to change a homosexual orientation to a heterosexual one. The evolution of one branch of psychoanalytic theory into an antihomosexual political movement illustrates the permeability of boundaries between clinical issues and political ones. The deletion of homosexuality from the *Diagnostic and Statistical Manual* has led to increased political activism and a rightward swing of reparative therapists. In removing the diagnostic label of illness, antihomosexual political, religious and mental health forces were deprived of an important tool of repression. The growing political activism of reparative therapists underscores how much actual repression was previously wrought by the diagnostic label itself. In their open support of antigay legislation, reparative therapists have moved from the traditional psychoanalytic center and have been embraced by conservative religious and political forces opposed to homosexuality. In doing so, they have apparently adopted religious organizational practices themselves, preaching dogma and stifling dissent. The increasing marginalization of reparative therapists from the psychoanalytic mainstream illustrates how psychoanalysis *per se* is neither gay-affirming nor condemning, although psychoanalytic practitioners may fall into either of these categories.

NOTES

1. Although this volume was published toward the end of his life, it is based on ideas and lectures that Rado developed and taught in the 1930s and 40s.

2. The American Psychiatric Association issued its first anti-discrimination statement on December 15, 1973. The American Academy of Psychoanalysis issued a non-discrimination statement in 1990. The American Psychoanalytic Association issued one in 1991.

3. With acknowledgment of the contributions of David Smith, M.D. at a presentation comparing the language of reparative therapists and religious fundamentalists at the 1995 meeting of the American Psychiatric Association, Miami, FL.

REFERENCES

Abelove, H. (1986), Freud, male homosexuality, and the Americans. In: *The Lesbian and Gay Studies Reader,* ed. H. Abelove, M.A. Barale, & D. Halperin. New York, NY: Routledge, 1993, pp. 381-393.

Bayer, R. (1981), *Homosexuality and American Psychiatry: The Politics of Diagnosis.* New York, NY: Basic Books.

Bieber, I., Dain, H., Dince, P., Drellich, M., Grand, H., Gundlach, R., Kremer, M., Rifkin, A., Wilbur, C. & Bieber T. (1962), *Homosexuality: A Psychoanalytic Study.* New York, NY: Basic Books.

Bullough, V. (1979), *Homosexuality: A History.* New York, NY: Meridian.

D'Ercole, A. (1996), Postmodern ideas about gender and sexuality: The lesbian woman redundancy, *Psychoanal. and Psychother.*, 13(2):142-152.

Domenici, T. & Lesser, R., ed. (1995), *Disorienting Sexuality: Psychoanalytic Reappraisals of Sexual Identities.* New York, NY: Routledge.

Drescher, J. (1995), Anti-homosexual bias in training. In: *Disorienting Sexuality*, ed. T. Domenici & R. Lesser, pp. 227-241. New York, NY: Routledge.

Drescher, J. (1996a), Psychoanalytic subjectivity and male homosexuality. In: *Textbook of Homosexuality and Mental Health.* ed. R. Cabaj & T. Stein, pp. 173-189. Washington, D.C.: American Psychiatric Press.

Drescher, J. (1996b), A discussion across sexual orientation and gender boundaries: Reflections of a gay male analyst to a heterosexual female analyst, *Gend. & Psychoanal.*, 1(2):223-237.

Drescher, J. (1997), From preoedipal to postmodern: Changing psychoanalytic attitudes toward homosexuality, *Gend. & Psychoanal*, 2(2): 203-216.

Drescher, J. (1998a), Contemporary psychoanalytic psychotherapy with gay men: With a commentary on reparative therapy of homosexuality. *J. of Gay and Lesbian Psychother.*, 2(4):51-74.

Drescher, J. (1998b), *Psychoanalytic Psychotherapy and The Gay Man*. Hillsdale, NJ: The Analytic Press.

Duberman, M. (1991), *Cures: A Gay Man's Odyssey*. New York, NY: Dutton.

Dunlap, D. (1995), An analyst, a father, battles homosexuality, *The New York Times*, December 24.

Freud, S. (1905), Three essays on the theory of sexuality. *Standard Edition*, 7:123-246. London: Hogarth Press, 1953.

Freud, S. (1908), "Civilized" sexual morality and modern mental illness. *Standard Edition*, 9:177-204. London: Hogarth Press, 1959.

Freud, S. (1909), Analysis of a phobia in a five-year-old boy. *Standard Edition*, 10:1-149. London: Hogarth Press, 1955.

Freud, S. (1910), Leonardo da Vinci and a memory of his childhood. *Standard Edition*, 11:59-138. London: Hogarth Press, 1957.

Freud, S. (1911), Psycho-analytic notes on an autobiographical account of a case of paranoia. *Standard Edition*, 12:1-82. London: Hogarth Press, 1958.

Freud, S. (1914), On narcissism: An introduction. *Standard Edition*, 14:73-102. London: Hogarth Press, 1957.

Freud, S. (1918), Lines of advance in psycho-analytic therapy. *Standard Edition*, 17:157-168. London: Hogarth Press, 1955.

Freud, S. (1920), The psychogenesis of a case of homosexuality in a woman. *Standard Edition*, 18:221-232. London: Hogarth Press, 1955.

Freud, S. (1923), Some neurotic mechanisms in jealousy, paranoia and homosexuality. *Standard Edition*, 18:145-172. London: Hogarth Press, 1955.

Freud, S. (1926), Inhibitions, symptoms and anxiety. *Standard Edition*, 20: 75-175. London: Hogarth Press, 1959.

Freud, S. (1935), Anonymous (Letter to an American mother). In: *The Letters of Sigmund Freud,* ed. E. Freud, 1960. New York, NY: Basic Books, pp. 423-424.

Gay, P. (1987), *A Godless Jew: Freud, Atheism and the Making of Psychoanalysis*. New Haven, CT: Yale University Press.

Glassgold, J. & Iasenza, S., ed. (1995), *Lesbians and Psychoanalysis: Revolutions in Theory and Practice*. New York, NY: The Free Press.

Greenberg J. and Mitchell S. (1983), *Object Relations in Psychoanalytic Theory*. Cambridge, MA: Harvard University Press.

Hamer, D. & Copeland, P. (1994), *The Science of Desire*. New York, NY: Simon & Schuster.

Isay, R. (1989), *Being Homosexual: Gay Men and Their Development*. New York, NY: Farrar, Straus and Giroux.

Isay, R. (1996), *Becoming Gay: The Journey to Self-Acceptance*. New York, NY: Pantheon.

Kardiner, A. (1955), *Sex and Morality*. London: Routledge and Kegan Paul LTD.

Kiersky, S. (1996), Exiled desire: The problem of reality in psychoanalysis and lesbian experience, *Psychoanal. and Psychother.*, 13(2):130-141.

Krafft-Ebing, R. (1886), *Psychopathia Sexualis*, trans. H. Wedeck. New York, NY: Putnam.

LeVay, S. (1993), *The Sexual Brain*. Cambridge, MA: The MIT Press.

Lewes, K. (1988), *The Psychoanalytic Theory of Male Homosexuality*. New York, NY: Simon and Schuster. Reissued as *Psychoanalysis and Male Homosexuality* (1995), Aronson.

Mahler, M., Pine, F. & Bergman, A. (1975), *The Psychological Birth of the Human Infant: Symbiosis and Individuation*. New York, NY: Basic Books.

Marrow, J. (1996), New wine, old bottle. *The Lesbian Review of Books*, 2(4): 13-14.

McWilliams, N. (1996), Therapy across the sexual orientation boundary: Reflections of a heterosexual female analyst on working with lesbian, gay and bisexual patients, *Gend. & Psychoanal.*, 1(2):203-221.

Nagourney, A. (1995), Father doesn't know best. *Out Magazine*, Feb., pp. 75-77, 113-115.

National Association for Research and Therapy of Homosexuality (1996), *Letter to Ralph Roughton, M.D. from Joseph Nicolosi, NARTH Secretary*, June 10.

National Conference of Catholic Bishops (1982), *Norms for Priestly Formation*. Washington, DC: United States Catholic Conference.

Nicolosi, J. (1991), *Reparative Therapy of Male Homosexuality: A New Clinical Approach*. Northvale, NJ: Aronson.

O'Connor, N. & Ryan, J. (1993), *Wild Desires and Mistaken Identities: Lesbianism & Psychoanalysis*. New York, NY: Columbia University.

Ovesey, L. (1969), *Homosexuality and Pseudohomosexuality*. New York, NY: Science House.

Rado, S. (1969), *Adaptational Psychodynamics: Motivation and Control*. New York, NY: Science House.

Roazen, P. & Swerdloff, B. (1995) *Heresy: Sandor Rado and the Psychoanalytic Movement*. Northvale, NJ: Aronson.

Socarides, C. (1968), *The Overt Homosexual*. New York, NY: Grune & Stratton.

Socarides, C. (1978), *Homosexuality*. New York, NY: Jason Aronson.

Socarides, C. (1993), District Court, City and Country of Denver, Colorado. Case No. 92 CV 7223. Affidavit of Charles W. Socarides, M.D. *Evans. v. Romer.*

Socarides, C. (1994a), Response to Judd Marmor, M.D. *Psychiatric News*, May 20.

Socarides, C. (1994b), The erosion of heterosexuality. *The Washington Times*, July 5.

Socarides, C. (1995), *Homosexuality: A Freedom Too Far*. Phoenix, AZ: Adam Margrave Books.

Socarides, C., Kaufman, B., Nicolosi, J., Satinover, J. & Fitzgibbons, R., (1997), Don't forsake homosexuals who want help. *The Wall Street Journal*, January 9.

Tiffen, L. (1994), *Creationism's Upside-Down Pyramid: How Science Refutes Fundamentalism*. Amherst, NY: Prometheus Books.

Wortis, J. (1954), *Fragments of an Analysis With Freud*. New York, NY: Charter Books.

The View from Irving Bieber's Couch: "Heads I Win, Tails You Lose"

Paul Moor

SUMMARY. The author recalls details of how he began and pursued a psychoanalytic treatment with the late Irving Bieber, MD. Having undergone an unsuccessful attempt to change his homosexual orientation, the author describes what he felt are some of the harmful consequences of that experience. *[Article copies available for a fee from The Haworth Document Delivery Service: 1-800-HAWORTH. E-mail address: <getinfo@ haworthpressinc.com> Website: <http://www.HaworthPress.com>]*

KEYWORDS. Irving Bieber, homosexuality, patient harm, psychoanalysis, reparative therapy, sexual conversion therapy

In March 2000, when the Board of Trustees of the American Psychiatric Association's Commission on Psychotherapy by Psychiatrists (COPP) approved a new position statement on reparative or conversion therapy for homosexual patients, one phrase leapt off the page at me: "[The] APA recommends that ethical practitioners refrain from attempts to change individuals' sexual orientation, keeping in mind the medical dictum to First, do no harm" (APA, 2000, p. 1719). More than half a century prior to that, cruel fate–plus sheer coincidence–had landed me on the couch of a New York psychoanalyst, my worst enemy might well have chosen for me. I refer to Irving Bieber, MD (1891-1991), who during his prime held a professorship of psychiatry at New

---

Paul Moor is a writer living and working in Berlin, Germany.

[Haworth co-indexing entry note]: "The View from Irving Bieber's Couch: 'Heads I Win, Tails You Lose.' " Moor, Paul. Co-published simultaneously in *Journal of Gay & Lesbian Psychotherapy* (The Haworth Medical Press, an imprint of The Haworth Press, Inc.) Vol. 5, No. 3/4, 2001, pp. 25-36; and: *Sexual Conversion Therapy: Ethical, Clinical and Research Perspectives* (ed: Ariel Shidlo, Michael Schroeder, and Jack Drescher) The Haworth Medical Press, an imprint of The Haworth Press, Inc., 2001, pp. 25-36. Single or multiple copies of this article are available for a fee from The Haworth Document Delivery Service [1-800-HAWORTH, 9:00 a.m. - 5:00 p.m. (EST). E-mail address: getinfo@haworthpressinc.com].

York Medical College in Valhalla as well as the office of President of the American Academy of Psychoanalysis. It took me not years but decades to realize the full extent of the harm he did to me during the nine months I was in "treatment" with him. During that time, I tied myself into psychological knots in my misguided attempts to adapt to his expectations and preconditions. These he imposed, I readily concede, with probably the best will in the world, for ironically, in every other respect, I will always remember him as a sincerely good man. If his medical accreditation included swearing allegiance to the Hippocratic Oath, he remained faithful to such passages as "I will use treatment to help the sick according to my ability and judgment, but never with a view to injury and wrongdoing . . . and I will abstain from all intentional wrongdoing and harm. . . . " Tragically, in that analyst's case, his ability and judgment entailed appallingly destructive wrongheadedness.

In retrospect it seems to me a minor miracle that my fundamental faith in psychoanalysis managed to survive that ordeal; after a hiatus of eleven years, which included my moving residence from New York to Europe, I did go on to two subsequent German analysts (the first of whom died, necessitating the third installment) in the hope of sorting out emotional problems to the utmost of my ability. After my first book appeared in Germany in 1972,[1] it attracted attention in psychoanalytic circles sufficiently favorable to gain me admittance to two psychoanalytic institutes in Berlin for what they called "informatory" training–all theoretical but no clinical or technical seminars. I feel my seven years of such training has enabled me to assess my own personal couch experiences retrospectively with rather more than average lay clarity and sophistication.

In 1962, fourteen years after I mustered the courage to remove myself from his personal conception of psychoanalysis and therapy, Bieber published a study with a team of U.S. analysts that swiftly and firmly established him as a leading crusader for what is today referred to as reparative or conversion therapy (Bieber et al., 1962). However, when I went to him for my first analysis in New York, I knew nothing about his opinions on homosexuality. Towards the end of World War II, through a mutual friend, I had met and very much liked his wife Toby Bieber. Soon after, when Dr. Bieber returned from military service to reopen his Manhattan practice, I met him at a party given at the home of that same friend. In good American fashion, I knew my future analyst on a first-name basis from the beginning. That period found me, in my early twenties, in considerable emotional distress and conflict, urgently in need of help. I had never before come into any kind of contact with any psychoanalyst, and my second encounter with Irving, in his office, involved the preliminary discussion leading to our third encounter, when I first took my place on his couch. He needed little time before making clear to me his firm opinion that he classified all homosexuals *ipso facto* as sick.

Even well before puberty, personal introspection had made my own homosexual inclinations unequivocally clear; adolescence made them almost overwhelmingly unmistakable and forceful. At age eighteen, my choice of friends attracted the attention of my older sister, a staff member of the university I attended. After a candid talk she pointed me in the direction of my first psychotherapeutic help: three fairly brief and superficial sessions with a University Health Service psychiatrist. He had nothing better to offer than the suggestion that I utilize my reasonably broad-minded sister as what he called "a buffer" between me and our Southern Baptist parents. I had two serious love affairs with men–one with a brilliant young music professor in mortal terror of being detected with a 17-year-old student–before I received my bachelor's degree at nineteen. Both affairs ended in a hurtful manner that left me feeling desperate and almost hopeless.[2] I naively regarded my homosexual nature itself, rather than my unfortunate choice of male partners, as the cause of my almost suicidal despondency. By the time I eventually went to Irving Bieber, I had one fundamental unequivocal petition: "Cure me. Heal me."

Once our sessions began, I cannot recall today how long he waited before confronting me with a fundamental postulate of his, which struck me from the beginning as utterly illogical. "Homosexual relations have as their foundation not love but hostility." I immediately got his message that I had to accept and adapt if I wanted to get the fullest possible benefit from my unfolding analysis. The shock of that proclamation so ambushed me that only a good deal later did Bieber's fundamental standpoint on homosexuality really get through to me: he categorically rejected the very idea of an emotionally and psychically healthy homosexual. For him, the very phrase "healthy homosexual" comprised an insoluble oxymoron. By all logic, I ought to have broken off our contacts then and there–but as the famous (and gay) novelist Somerset Maugham once so pithily put it, "Most of us become writers because we can never think of the apt thing to say till the moment to say it has past."[3]

I concede that since Bieber's sweeping proclamation about hostility as an *Ersatz* for love I have indeed observed not a few relationships–hetero- as well as homosexual–held together less by love than what Robert Stoller (1975) once deftly labeled "the erotic form of hatred." However, even at that age, I already knew what I would subsequently learn from a major relationship: no one, not even Bieber, could legitimately classify as "hostility" the profoundly affectionate, warm, life-enhancing emotion I felt for men with whom I have fallen in love–as deeply as anyone could ever fall in love with anyone. In retrospect, what Bieber stipulated as my adjustment to his therapy amounted to as violent a *volte-face* as Orwell's "Newspeak" or "Newthink": "War Is Peace, Hate Is Love," and so on. I wish I had realized it at the time, but I didn't. The invisible man watching me from the head of his couch felt to me like a somewhat less baleful psychoanalytic version of Big Brother.

For example, at every possible opportunity Irving would repeat–more times than I could even begin to estimate–one sentence I gradually came to antici-pate with an inner wince: "There is no shortage of beautiful women." On the one occasion he ever varied that refrain, it came as a minor shock to hear, "There is no shortage of lovely women." Obviously he expected the pitiless repetition of that mantra to have a therapeutic effect upon me; it had, in fact, the familiar effect of water on a duck's back.[4] Even by the time I discontinued my sessions with him, that litany had had no more effect on me than it had the first time he trotted it out.

Another oft-repeated proclamation was, "Your sexuality is no different from any other man's." I mulled that over for a long time, unsuccessfully, be-fore finally working up the courage to challenge him with "What do you mean, the same–you know as well as I do that only men attract me sexually." To that kind of rejoinder he always tried the soothing assurance (the unuttered phrase "Trust me" hung in the air) that really and truly, deep, deep down inside me, there lay some bedrock truth he magically knew. It was a truth he claimed to know far better than I myself; and in time he expected to reveal it to me, if only I would exert myself sufficiently to follow the path he prescribed. This set me up for the reparative therapist's treacherous fundamental assumption: if, in spite of all his expert treatment and his wholly sincere efforts to straighten me out, I obstinately remained attracted to men, then I, not he, had failed. I alone would bear the burden of responsibility for that delinquency. It was my own disinclination to face up to and admit such a crushing defeat that kept me re-turning to his couch a good deal longer than I otherwise would have.

I tried–God knows I tried!–to give him what he wanted. However, those at-tempts of mine to get something started with a member of the opposite sex re-peatedly landed me in situations far more embarrassing and painful than any third person, analyst or not, could ever have imagined. Repeated experience had taught me I could pass as straight with almost all the people who knew me, yet my camouflage stood me in no stead at all with more than one bright young woman I hesitantly approached as potentially exploitable to me in my hetero-sexual undertaking. I would sum up their consistent reactions as quizzical at best–and excruciatingly humiliating at worst.

Almost inevitably, they knew enough about the sexual facts of life to size me up correctly, no matter how otherwise effective my external camouflage. That in itself hurt deeply enough, but it hurt almost unendurably if they took the additional step of telling me their candid conclusion–for they thus con-fronted me with raw refutation of what Dr. Bieber so sincerely wanted to be-come true. Any manifestation of any kind of impotence embarrasses almost any man, and that situation, especially when it materialized during such an early stage, embarrassed and hurt me almost beyond the power of words to de-scribe. The fact that impotence had never clouded any of my sexual contacts with a man merely compounded my desperation. It only too forcefully reminded me of the formidable obstacle Irving told me I had ahead of me, which I would have to overcome in order to attain the goal I had my heart set on when I first came to him as a patient.

A few months into my treatment with Bieber had passed when a neighbor of mine, affiliated with Alfred C. Kinsey's sex research team, told me Dr. Kinsey had come to New York. He was there in connection with one of his later specialized studies of specific population groups, in this instance artists, and Kinsey would like to take my history, specifically as a musician. With me still in my early twenties, such attention from such a celebrity flattered me into assenting, so one afternoon I went by appointment to tell all to the great man in his room at mid-Manhattan's Hotel Pennsylvania. Fairly early in our exchange, I told him that I had begun psychoanalysis and that I hoped to lick the homosexuality that had caused me so much unhappiness for about half my life. "Do you feel you've made progress in that direction?" "Yes"–my own truth at that moment, thanks to the unrelenting repetitiveness of those sessions on Irving Bieber's couch. Kinsey sounded sincere when he made his only comment: "I'm delighted to hear it."

The questionnaire took several hours and the end brought a dispassionate, factual summary from Kinsey. My uniquely experienced interlocutor made the following shattering appraisal, "You say psychoanalysis has helped you progress in the direction of heterosexuality. However, on the basis of your entire history of sexual behavior, I would have to categorize you as either a six or at most a five"– and I already knew that on the famous Kinsey (Kinsey et al., 1948) scale of human sexual behavior, "six" meant exclusively homosexual and "five" meant almost, but not quite, exclusively homosexual. Even more crushingly, Kinsey told me that neither he nor his team, during all those years they had spent taking thousands of histories, had ever found one authentic instance of sexual repolarization as determined on the basis of dreams, fantasies, and genital response. Hearing that from Dr. Kinsey himself did force me to recognize an undeniable truth I had done my level best to repress and deny. I had done so to avoid disappointing my exalted analyst–who of course knew everything and whom I desperately wanted to please. However, my belief that Kinsey knew more about human sexual behavior than anybody else on earth had an electrifying but also depressing effect upon me, specifically with regard to my very motivation for going into analysis.

At my next session with Irving, naturally I reported Kinsey's assessment. I could not see my analyst's face, but his voice transmitted his intense irritation. He must have immediately recognized what a major setback that verdict from such a unique expert had to mean from my own perspective. I cannot say he sputtered exactly, but I can say that his voiced efforts to counteract Kinsey's dicta, and get me pointed back in the straight direction, struck me as unconvincing and intellectually less than honest. This was indeed a disturbing discovery to make in the person to whom I had so unconditionally entrusted so much.

The beginning of the end of my analysis with Irving came during the months following a Christmastide introduction to the music editor of an important national newsmagazine that swiftly led to a promising intimate relationship. It was so reciprocally compatible–we had so many mutual interests, so many, many things and friends in common–that at his own suggestion, for all practical purposes, I soon virtually moved in with him. My promising new lover and I remained as happy and harmonious as ever. Then Irving, with no warning, proclaimed the way things would have to go, as of right then. The time had come, he decreed, when in the interest of my analysis I would have to set aside this new homosexual relationship and devote myself with completely focused concentration towards reinforcing the heterosexual component of my nature.

Such a proclamation, handed down like a Mosaic table of the law, left me speechless for a long moment. When he saw that I intended to balk, he persisted: "Isn't that what you told me you wanted most of all the first day you came here to see me?" And there, of course, he had me. Now, however, came my own turn to sputter: "But . . . but . . . your *ordering* me to do such a thing hardly conforms with what I've always heard about conventional psychoanalysis." With audible equanimity: "Did I ever tell you I was a conventional analyst?" And there, of course, he had me again, at least figuratively, by the balls. I can no longer recall how many more times I continued to go to him after that, but that pivotal session marked the beginning of the end. My important new personal relationship still seemed to promise so much that I had no intention of sacrificing it merely to conform to Irving Bieber's strictly theoretical outsider assumption concerning my innermost nature.

That troubled period brought additional complications in my life, topped by my losing the script-writing job that had officially turned me, at the age of twenty, into a professional writer. I had borrowed a considerable sum to buttress my own ability to pay for my analytic sessions. In those blessed days Irving charged five dollars an hour–but even that fee placed a prohibitive strain upon the fifty dollars a week my job paid me. After I lost my job, I reluctantly had to go into debt with Irving. After fifty-two years I can no longer say for certain, but I believe both my financial setback and my unwillingness to end my relationship constituted a turning-point that left me under no illusion as to where I stood with him as an uncooperative patient. From the beginning of the analysis, Irving had assigned me three regular hours a week; they belonged to me and me alone. Now, suddenly, he told me, at the end of each hour, some completely different time for my next hour, two or three days later. This left me feeling that he had demoted me in rank among his patients and that I was being subjected to indirect punishment for my recalcitrance: either come at this new time, and on comparably short notice, or else. . . . What with one thing and another, Irving eventually broke the news to me that my allotting first priority to my new lover meant that we should at least interrupt therapy–which never did get resumed.[5]

Curiously enough, that break did not bring an end to all contact between Irving Bieber and me. The Biebers and I had originally met socially, I had known and liked Toby for quite some time before I became Irving's patient, and at least on a considerably diminished scale those purely social contacts did continue, on a more or less annual basis after my move to Europe in 1949. After I reestablished contact on a social level with him and Toby (and I hastily pass over the phenomenon of an analyst's marrying a woman with that traditionally masculine name–the only instance I have ever known of a female Toby), for a period of many years I continued to see them on our original pre-analysis social level.

Even prior to that, during my analysis, I recall several encounters I believe would bring a frown to most analysts' faces. Preparing a piano recital, I invited a couple of women friends to my place one evening for a trial run of my program–and since they belonged to the same circle where I'd first met Irving, and since I knew Toby had gone out of town, I offhandedly asked him whether he might like to come, too, and to my considerable surprise he did. That evening at my apartment he remained fairly taciturn, but I do recall my less than comfortable impression of his studying me, as though on a sort of peripheral psychoanalytic field-trip.[6]

Such bi-stratal contacts with Irving–both with and without Toby, both during and after my months of analysis with him–left me curiously off-balance as to the fundamental nature of our extant relationship. For at least eleven years he remained the only psychoanalyst, anywhere in the world, to whom I had any kind of contact. Even after my 1949 move to Europe, I more often than not checked in socially with "Irv and Tobe," as they called each other, when I returned to the USA at almost annual intervals. This, in turn, usually led to a meeting for lunch or dinner, sometimes in their apartment. On one such evening, when Irving let me in and spent several minutes with me before Toby came in from her own treatment room, I still recall how it took me aback a bit when she came right at me with a warm welcoming smile and extended arms and a cordial "Let's have a hug!"[7]

It was during one of those social visits that I spoke to Irving about C.A. Tripp, a psychologist who, in 1975, published *The Homosexual Matrix*. There he wrote:

> . . . [The] Kinsey Research made a concerted effort over a period of years
> to find and evaluate the histories of people whose sex lives had changed

either during or following therapy of any kind. None was ever found. Several psychoanalysts who were friends of the Research promised to send particular patients they were proud of having 'cured,' but none of these was ever forthcoming. After Kinsey's death, and to this day, Wardell Pomeroy . . . has maintained a standing offer to administer the Kinsey Research battery to any person a therapist might send, and thus possibly validate a case of changed homosexuality. This offer has never had any 'takers' except for one remarkable instance.

A New York psychiatrist who for a number of years has headed a large psychoanalytic research program on homosexuality–a man who has written an important book on the subject in which various percentages of changed cases were reported–did indeed make a definite commitment to exemplify these results. After several delays of several weeks each the psychiatrist finally confessed to Pomeroy that he had only one case which he thought would qualify but that, unfortunately, he was on such bad terms with the patient he did not feel free to call him up.

Tripp, although he did not mention him by name, called Irving's work a "misrepresentation." Bieber subsequently filed a formal ethics complaint against Tripp with the American Psychological Association in which he accused him of impugning his "scientific honesty and credibility." However, the APA decided there was no evidence of unethical behavior on Tripp's part and he was exonerated.

I read about the details of Bieber's complaint in the second, 1987 edition of Tripp's book. Armed with such belated intelligence, I asked Irving at our next encounter, during one of my New York visits with him, whether he had maintained follow-up contact with the patients that he and his colleagues claimed had successfully made the transition from homo- to heterosexuality. His answer consisted of an unqualified "no"–and during the pause that followed he offered no elaboration. Unavoidably, that adds up to an admission of no evidence whatever concerning the durability of those reorientations he and his team claimed.

Nevertheless, Irving Bieber remained inflexibly faithful to his contentions until the day he died. *The New York Times'* fairly lengthy obituary[8] included the unqualified statement that "he was best known for his controversial view of homosexuality. He believed it was an illness that could be treated or prevented through psychotherapy–a view that has since been discredited." Period. The obituary went on to say:

> Dr. Bieber's study helped bring candor to the discussion of homosexuality, but his view of it as deviant behavior was controversial even then and has since been disavowed. In 1973, the American Psychiatric Association removed homosexuality from its list of psychiatric disorders, but Dr.

Bieber remained steadfast, telling an interviewer the same year that "a homosexual is a person whose heterosexual function is crippled, like the legs of a polio victim."

I feel slightly uneasy about writing what some might dismiss as delayed Oedipal retribution, for I long ago discovered that one of the greatest tragedies in *conditio humana* derives from the fact that everyone–everyone–has his reasons. I don't for a moment doubt that Irving Bieber regarded me with affection and wanted only the best for me. Unfortunately, and tragically, that does not alter the dominant reality that his intended good did me in fact literally irreparable harm, which it took me not years but decades to realize fully–and at least partially repair, to a considerable extent by self-analysis. That reality also motivates my now doing everything in my power to prevent his inhumane kind of reparative or conversion therapy from wreaking similar harm upon troubled "homosexuals" who in my wake have also sought help in psychotherapy.

So two fundamental question remains: What harm did Irving Bieber's concept of therapy do me and what harm does it continue to do? There is one residue of Dr. Bieber's therapy which I carried with me for so long. As a lover of words and a professional devotee to their precise meanings, I for many years had the greatest difficulty even using the term "gay" as the prevalent synonym for "homosexual." In my own experience, I had found little about life as a homosexual that I could conscientiously call "gay." While living in the free and easy atmosphere of the world's gay capital, San Francisco, that tacit aversion constantly forced me to make evasive conversational detours. I know I must have seriously annoyed San Francisco's gay Supervisor Harry Britt, first the adjutant and then the direct successor to the great gay activist pioneer Harvey Milk, when during an interview with him it became painfully obvious that I simply could not use that crucial word the way he did. The attrition of daily life in San Francisco finally wore me down, but not until I read Richard Isay's books *Being Homosexual: Gay Men and Their Development* (1989) and *Becoming Gay: The Journey to Self-Acceptance* (1996) did the true semantic and psychological connotations of that term become clear to me–and move me finally to capitulate to *force majeure*. Now in my 77th year, I look back with profound regret at innumerable instances when things would have worked out more happily. However, a well-intentioned but horribly misguided man left an almost indelible impression upon me more than half a century ago.

To begin with, Irving Bieber had successfully instilled into me the cruelly wrong belief that the more I yielded to my virtually irresistible attraction towards men–for me the most natural thing in the world–the more I would simply prolong my own self-destructive torment. I do indeed blame him for having so cruelly perverted my own essential attitude towards my own sexuality. The psychological damage in my early childhood had begun with the numerous pathological inhibitions I knew as part and parcel of family life, inculcated by parents disastrously unsuited for each other. It was added to by the unquestioning fervor of both parents' acceptance of the puritanical Southern Baptist Convention that branded all extra-marital sex as evil, with same-sex activity the evillest of all. Far from helping me recover from that inhumane perversion of my basic innermost drives and needs, Irving Bieber in large and important measure reinforced those pathologically perverting strictures as a convenient potential implement to prove his own abstract theories.

Probably worst of all–and for not years but decades–Irving Bieber's residual malefaction left me in a variation of the classic, quintessential double bind: if I, as an emotionally sick and suffering patient, desperately eager to please my certified and psychically healthy expert guru, did what he wanted me to do, that meant I would have to repress, deny, and somehow even overcome, oppose, and counteract the most powerful vital urge that came most naturally to me. If I failed to do that, for no matter what reason, then not he but I had erred and would forever personally have to bear the responsibility for that failure.

Heads, I win; tails, you lose.

Irving Bieber had this crack-brained, unshakable conviction that towards the male objects of my affections I really and truly felt not love but hostility. For many years that belief which he inculcated in me hung like a miasma over my relations with men, with me recurrently bothered by preposterous self-scrutiny. Did Dr. Bieber's specialized wisdom correctly recognize and explain the spontaneous emotions I felt so strongly within me, which in my lay ignorance I so stupidly mistook for affection, even love? Instead, his early indoctrination left me, for so unnecessarily and avoidably protracted a period of years, a member of that category the military so aptly categorize as the walking wounded. As so often since then, in connection with that specific situation and a few others like it, I think of John Greenleaf Whittier's couplet:

> For of all sad words of tongue or pen,
> The saddest are these: "It might have been."

NOTES

1. *Das Selbstporträt des Jürgen Bartsch* (Fischer Taschenbuch Verlag, Frankfurt)–after his death vastly expanded into *Jürgen Bartsch: Opfer und Täter* (Rowohlt Verlag, Hamburg/Reinbek, 1991).

2. During that time I also became involved in the most protracted of my very few heterosexual affairs, but the initiative came totally from my partner, who was nine years older than I.

3. Introduction to *The Portable Dorothy Parker* (The Viking Press, New York, 1944), p. 12.

4. Even my comparatively superficial subsequent Berlin institutional training made me aware of a number of flagrant unorthodoxies on Irving's part that hardly facilitated my making any real progress with him.

5. As a non-analyst I hesitate even to touch upon the prickly question of psychoanalysts and money, but there is one fiscal postscript I do find worth mentioning for the light it may cast upon Irving Bieber's reaction concerning the debt I had accumulated with him in order to continue analysis. Some years later, with my finances improved, I raised the subject of my debt with him–and he dismissed it with a wave of the hand: "Forget it."

6. Almost thirty years ago, in conversation, when I questioned one world-famous analyst I knew personally about some fairly outrageous unorthodoxy on his own part that had come to my attention, he told me smoothly: "A good analyst can do anything as long as he knows what he's doing"–to which I riposted: "Have you ever known any analyst who didn't consider himself a good analyst?" In other words, according to that self-serving pseudo-logic, which may not apply to all analysts but assuredly did to Bieber, any analyst has *carte blanche* to do anything . . . and the hapless patient take the hindmost.

7. Not until years later would I learn the extent to which Toby and Irving Bieber saw eye to eye on me and my perverted ilk. At one time she served as a faculty member of New York Medical College, and belonged to the group-therapy faculty of the Contemporary Center for Advanced Psychoanalytic Studies in New Jersey. One excerpt from her own writing will suffice: "In nearly thirty years, I have successfully concluded analyses of one hundred homosexuals . . . and have seen nearly five hundred cases in consultation. . . . On the basis of the experience thus gathered, I make the positive statement that homosexuality has an excellent prognosis in psychiatric-psychoanalytic treatment of one to two years' duration, with a minimum of three appointments each week–provided the patient really wishes to change . . . " (Bieber, 1971, p. 532). Note that facile all-purpose escape hatch: if the patient at the end of that time remains recalcitrantly homosexual, the true wish to change had simply proved insufficient.

8. My twinge of knee-jerk residual *Schadenfreude* surprised me when I discovered a photograph of another man attached to Irving's obituary.

REFERENCES

American Psychiatric Association (2000), Commission on Psychotherapy by Psychiatrists (COPP): Position statement on therapies focused on attempts to change sexual orientation (Reparative or conversion therapies). *Amer. J. Psychiat.*, 157:1719-1721.

Bieber, I., Dain, H., Dince, P., Drellich, M., Grand, H., Gundlach, R., Kremer, M., Rifkin, A., Wilbur, C., & Bieber T. (1962), *Homosexuality: A Psychoanalytic Study*. New York: Basic Books.

Bieber, T. (1971), Group therapy with homosexuals. In: *Comprehensive Group Psychotherapy*, eds. H. I. Kaplan & B. J. Sadock. Baltimore, MD: Williams and Wilkins.

Isay, R. (1989), *Being Homosexual: Gay Men and Their Development*. New York: Farrar, Straus and Giroux.

Isay, R. (1996), *Becoming Gay: The Journey to Self-Acceptance.* New York: Pantheon.

Kinsey, A., Pomeroy, W., & Martin, C. (1948), *Sexual Behavior in the Human Male.* Philadelphia, PA: Saunders.

Myers, S. L. (1991), Irving Bieber, 80, a psychoanalyst who studied homosexuality, dies. *The New York Times,* August 28.

Stoller, R. (1975), *Perversion: The Erotic Form of Hatred.* New York: Pantheon Books.

Tripp, C. A. (1975), *The Homosexual Matrix.* New York: Meridian.

Excerpts
from *Cures: A Gay Man's Odyssey*

Martin Duberman, PhD

Historian Martin Duberman published a groundbreaking memoir in 1991, *Cures: A Gay Man's Odyssey*, in which, among other things, he chronicled his repeated attempts, as a young man, to try and change his sexual identity. His autobiographical account poignantly illustrates the subjectivity of many who engage in such struggles, while introducing readers to the individuals who claim to have the "cure." Duberman's most detailed description of his experiences in therapy was his last. As he put it, "This time–the last time–would prove far and away the most traumatic. It would involve five years of treatment that would take me to the brink not of reconstruction but of near-negation. It would so thoroughly undermine my ability to accept my own nature that . . . I would become nearly as homophobic as the culture itself." Interested readers should read *Cures* for themselves. Below are reprinted accounts of Duberman's earlier, briefer attempts to address his unwanted homosexual desires.

I

Duberman begins his memoir in 1948, just before his 18th birthday. During a rest stop on a cross-country biking trip, he goes to a fair in Calgary where he is enticed into the tent of Gemma, a gypsy fortune-teller:

Dr. Duberman is Distinguished Professor of History, City University of New York, Founder and First Director of CUNY's Center for Lesbian and Gay Studies, and a member of the *Journal of Gay & Lesbian Psychotherapy*'s editorial board.

Cures: A Gay Man's Odyssey, Tenth Anniversary Edition, with a new Preface and Afterword by the author is scheduled for release in April 2002 from Westview Press.

[Haworth co-indexing entry note]: "Excerpts from *Cures: A Gay Man's Odyssey*." Duberman, Martin. Co-published simultaneously in *Journal of Gay & Lesbian Psychotherapy* (The Haworth Medical Press, an imprint of The Haworth Press, Inc.) Vol. 5, No. 3/4, 2001, pp. 37-50; and: *Sexual Conversion Therapy: Ethical, Clinical and Research Perspectives* (ed: Ariel Shidlo, Michael Schroeder, and Jack Drescher) The Haworth Medical Press, an imprint of The Haworth Press, Inc., 2001, pp. 37-50. Single or multiple copies of this article are available for a fee from The Haworth Document Delivery Service [1-800-HAWORTH, 9:00 a.m. - 5:00 p.m. (EST). E-mail address: getinfo@haworthpressinc.com].

"I want you to write down"–seemingly from nowhere she produced a pad and pencil–"the one question that most preys on your mind. Do you understand?"

"I thought you already knew the question."

Gemma smiled enigmatically. "I feel I need to provide you with proof."

"One question?"

"Keep it brief. As short as possible. After writing down the question, fold the paper once and then place it under the piece of glass. Be sure to fold the paper over, so that the writing is not visible. After you have done that, I want you to sit back, close your eyes, and concentrate as deeply as possible on the question you have written down. I, too, shall close my eyes. I will empty my mind to receive your message. But you must concentrate very hard or you will not succeed in transmitting the message to me. Is that clear?"

"Wouldn't it be simpler if I just asked you the question?"

Again the enigmatic smile. "But then you would not believe that I have the power to read what is inside you without being told."

I wrote on the piece of paper, "Will I always be a homosexual?" Then, following her instructions, I folded the paper and put it under the crystal. But my skeptical side simply refused to sit back and concentrate. Not for the last time in encounters with my saviors, my rebellious side abruptly took over. I peeked. I saw Gemma take the piece of paper out through some opening in the bottom of the table, read it, then put it back.

"Open your eyes now," she said. "You are indeed a very troubled young man. Just as I had thought. But there is hope. Your particular trouble can be cured. But you must *want* to be cured"–a phrase I would hear often in the years ahead.

"What do you mean?"

"I mean you must give yourself up wholly to the cure. You must leave your old life, at once, and join our gypsy family so that I can be constantly by your side."

"Join your gypsy family?" The full absurdity of what Gemma was suggesting was clear. And yet, I *was* tempted–though I'd seen her trick with the paper, though my skepticism was entirely to the fore. I can still feel the powerful impulse within me to do exactly as she suggested. *Anything* to relieve the burden.

At least I was able to delay the decision. Fumbling toward the tent opening, I told Gemma I would have to think about it overnight, that in all likelihood I would do as she said, but that I first had to make "certain arrangements." As I walked out of her tent back on to the midway, she whispered gently, "It is your one chance for happiness"–another prediction I would hear often in the years ahead.

In the upshot, I did not appear at Gemma's tent at dawn, carrying my worldly goods. I went to Yale instead.

II

Having graduated from Yale and then gone on to graduate school at Harvard, Duberman recounts his early, adult sexual experiences and relationships, most of which were fraught with feelings of guilt, anxiety, and remorse. After the breakup of an affair with "Rob," he contemplates going into therapy:

I suppose I might have rushed right then and there into a psychiatrist's office. But one unpleasant memory and one wondrous new experience delayed that outcome for several years more. The memory was from age fifteen, when my parents had sent me to my first therapist. Knowing nothing of my sexual orientation, the "cure" they had sought was for my mysterious silence around the house (the mystery is less dense in retrospect; I was trying to avoid scrutiny and detection; the sense already having dawned in me that I had a desperate secret to hide). Monosyllabic at home, I was exuberantly verbal outside it, a gregarious leader among my friends. My parents knew that, deplored the contrast, blamed me for it, decided a therapist could "fix" it.

I saw the therapist for a few months, but never told him about my sexual attraction to other boys. I instinctively distrusted him, perhaps because of his paeans to the wonders of family life and filial duty, and his insistence that if I would regularly embrace my mother and tell her I loved her, all would come right. Once, in recounting a dream, I came perilously close to telling the therapist more than I intended. Masturbating to a homoerotic fantasy in a room enclosed by glass walls, I was terrified that people in nearby buildings would see what I was doing and discover the truth about me. "Which was what?" the therapist asked. "Dunno," I replied, quickly recovering my protective monosyllabism.

That happened seven or eight years before I met Rob: but the memory slowed my progress to the psychoanalytic couch. Anyway, I told myself, the failure of a mere affair was hardly sufficient proof that, as psychiatry would have it, I and all homosexuals were incapable of forming satisfying relationships. After all, even heterosexuals had brief, inconsequential affairs. And besides, the several good friendships I had formed of late certainly seemed to argue for my capacity to connect well with others.

But far more convincing proof of my intactness–and my lack of need for therapy–came along within a few months of the breakup with Rob; I fell in love. Nothing did more to make me willing to take up the onerous burden of a homosexual identity and to resist the psychiatric notion that *only* malediction would be my lot. Love felt a lot more like relief and joy.

III

At the age of twenty three, Duberman meets and falls in love with Larry:

We met at the Napoleon, a few months after I broke up with Rob. Larry was twenty, three years younger than I. He lived with his devoutly Catholic, working-class Irish family in Canton, a suburb outside of Boston, commuting every day to a clerk's job with Filene's department store (from which he gradually worked himself up to be a buyer). We were different in many ways besides class status. Larry was muscular and compact in build, low-keyed, intense, essentially nonverbal. He was my somatic ideal, I was his intellectual one; he helped me learn about my body, I helped him learn about books and ideas.

Though our differences were in some ways deeply nurturing, allowing us to open up new worlds for each other, we worried from the beginning that our pervasive differences in background, education, and temperament would ultimately overwhelm our passionate feelings of attachment and our sense that we did, profoundly and illogically, belong together.

We were expected to worry. And about much more than temperamental differences. Two people of the same gender, the culture had taught us, were not meant to spend their lives together and, should they be foolish enough to try, would soon learn that Nature intended otherwise. As if that conviction was not debilitating enough, we also had to cope (as did heterosexuals) with the then-current cultural nostrum that when two partners were *really* meant for each other, neither sexual arousal nor emotional commitment ever flagged; health was defined as the absence of desire for more than one person, or at least the need to act on the desire.

Larry and I didn't vary from the acceptable pattern for about two years. From the beginning, young and hot, our eyes strayed constantly. But we were under several spells–the mainstream American injunction to be faithful, love, and the fear of losing love–and they held our hormones in check. [One friend] constantly told us, his voice resonant with campy amazement, how *incredibly* lucky we were to have found each other and what *utter* ingrates we would be should we ever do *anything* to jeopardize our good fortune.

Properly chastised and warned, Larry and I scarcely dared think about outside sexual contacts, dutifully concentrating instead on the seemly issue of whether we should or could live together. Since we were both scraping by financially (I was now self-supporting, or at least trying to get by with minimal family assists), moving in together seemed a pipe dream for the time being. This was an impasse that carried with it some relief for me, since I still felt ambivalent, even if less so under the trance of love, about settling down as a now-and-forever homosexual. We made do with weekend overnights in my single bed (by 1954 I was a resident tutor in Adams House, with far more privacy than when living in the graduate school dormitory).

But by 1955, after Larry and I had been together for two years, amorous zest and fantasies of eternal togetherness began, in tandem, to fray a bit. As they do, of course, with most couples, romantic intensity inevitably mutating (when the couple is lucky) into a more routine and comfortable domesticity. It's also commonplace for partners to view any erosion in erotic excitement with alarm, as a forecast of ultimate disaster. But the forecast seems more ominous still when the couple consists of two gay men who have been forewarned of their incompatibility and told that sex was all they cared about and were good at anyway.

Larry and I continued to feel considerable passion for each other, but since it was no longer automatic and constant and now seemed to follow arguments rather than forestall them, we nervously wondered how much of a future we could count on. The more we wondered, the more prone we became to elevating garden-variety disagreements into the equivalent of Doomsday. And so we began to hedge our bets, slacken our commitment. (If it was only a matter of time before we broke up, maybe we ought to start looking around now for likely replacements?) Both of us, but I more than Larry, began having sexual adventures on the side. This deviation from the monogamous norm, in turn, further convinced me of my incapacity–generic, so long as I remained homosexual–for intimacy. Hadn't psychiatry long warned that homosexuals were condemned, by the very nature of their illness, to flee from relatedness to promiscuity?

Even if the culture had been supportive, Larry and I might have broken up; some of our differences, after all, did not bode well for the kind of long-term commitment that feeds best on companionable similarities of temperament and interest. But for straight couples, social values serve to counteract problems in the relationship; the high premium placed on heterosexual pair-bonding and family life provides plenty of brownie points and self-esteem for staying together. For homosexual couples, social values serve further to underscore, rather than counteract, interpersonal difficulties; being called "sick" and "degenerate" hardly gives one the needed psychic support for sustaining a relationship.

I began thinking once more about psychotherapy, thinking about "conversion" as my only hope for a happy life . . . I began seeing "Dr. Weintraupt" in late 1955, after the spiral of recrimination and reconciliation between Larry and me had come to seem hopelessly circular. These were the years when–for the privileged–and particularly for those living on the Eastern Seaboard, the decision to enter therapy seemed logical and valid. In a culture that had grown apolitical and conservative, analyzing the inner life had become a primary, praiseworthy enterprise. For intellectuals and egotists especially, it was the elective choice of the moment, *the* certified path to self knowledge.

From the first Weintraupt advised me to give up the relationship with Larry. Until I did, he warned, any real progress in therapy would prove impossible. The drama of our interpsychic struggle, Weintraupt insisted, had become a stand-in for the more basic intrapsychic conflict I was unwilling to engage–the conflict between my neurotic homosexual "acting out" and my underlying healthy impulse toward a heterosexual union.

I resisted–not so much Weintraupt's theories, as his insistence on a total break with Larry. I accepted the need, but could not summon the will. I spent therapy hour after therapy hour arguing my inability to give up the satisfactions of the relationship–neurotic and occasional though they might be, and though my future happiness might well hang on their surrender. I resisted so hard and long that Weintraupt finally gave me an ultimatum: either give up Larry or give up therapy.

September 10

[After several weeks of agonizing, Duberman writes in his diary,] I quit the analysis this morning. After months of indecision, the final action was almost unexpected. I told Weintraupt about last night with Larry [we had had sex]– and about a dream in which my "auditing" a course evolved into a symbolic reenactment of my attitude towards the analysis–i.e., an onlooker, an auditor, rather than a participant. From there it was only a step to being told my attitude made the analysis circular and endless; and since in honesty I couldn't swear that I would be able to change it, it was mutually agreed that it would be best to stop. Yet having made the decision, I can't accept it. Accepting it means accepting my life, being satisfied with it. And I can't . . .

I told Larry immediately about my decision to quit therapy, and we met for a serious talk about our future. We began the evening by having sex ("How great not to follow it," I wrote in my diary, "with panic and guilt"). Then later, over dinner, I told him that the best I thought I could manage would be a part-time relationship, no strings attached. I was happy, I said, for us to go on seeing each other–if he was–but no longer thought an exclusive relationship would work, explaining (as I wrote in my diary) that "I remain incapable (don't all homosexuals?) of finding satisfaction permanently with one person." Larry, an accepting stoic by nature, and extraordinarily tolerant of my mercurial shifts, asked for no further details or explanations and simply agreed henceforth to a loose arrangement between us.

But in a real sense, therapy had already poisoned that well. Weintraupt's certitudes about the hopelessness of homosexual life managed to underscore all my pre-existing doubts about my–or any homosexual's–capacity for love and commitment. Like most homosexual couples in those years, Larry and I had distrusted ourselves far too much to affirm what might have been genuinely different, and creatively different, about a gay relationship, to affirm (rather than apologize for) some needed distinctions between emotional and sexual fidelity. Instead we had invested our energies, as well as our hopes for certification as *bona fide* human beings, in conforming as closely as possible to the mainstream norm of what constituted a healthy union–meaning now-and-forever monogamy. Not the least of the sabotages the conformist fifties committed was to instill the notion that "different" was the equivalent of "disturbed" and, in the case of political nonconformists especially, "dangerous."

But being declared an unfit candidate for intimacy released me, ironically (though the irony escaped me at the time), better to enjoy the pleasures of the flesh. I was a horny young guy who had never before had license to explore the nonmonogamous urges of his body; being certified as "sick" hobbled my confidence but liberated my libido. I even had the occasional inkling that in breaking away from Larry I was *using* the insistence of orthodox psychiatry that I was incapacitated for love to justify some unorthodox and overdue sexual adventuring that the culture would sanction only for those lost souls unable to partake of the *real* satisfactions of monogamy.

I now began to roam with a vengeance, as if–being a dutiful creature of the culture–determined to live out Weintraupt's prediction that only therapy could have saved me from a life of random, disconnected promiscuity . . . I alternated between fits of remorse over quitting therapy ("throwing away my one chance at health") and self-recrimination over my inability either fully to commit or fully to withdraw from the relationship with Larry. He, within a few weeks, tried to bring matters to a head by putting a ban on our having sex ("We've got to try to form a new kind of relationship–friends, since lovers hasn't worked; and occasional sex with each other is merely postponing the adjustment"). Larry said he still preferred going to bed only with me, but rather than settle for occasionally, he had decided he preferred never–knowing the thought of never would frighten me more than him.

. . . Despite having broken off forever, within a short time we were again having sex. This time, more than a little exhausted at all the reformulations, we avoided cementing a pact of any kind and simply let our meetings take what shape they would. By now I was nearing completion of my doctoral thesis, and both Larry and I knew that within a year I would be leaving the Boston area for a full-time teaching job. We no longer had any expectation about sharing our lives in the future–though there would be occasional pangs of longing and regret for several more years, and for several decades (for we did stay in touch) unexpected surges of deep feeling for each other.

When I took up my first teaching job at Yale in the fall of 1957, Larry and I still occasionally alternated weekends in Boston or New Haven. Saying good-bye to him after one of them, I remember tears gushing from my eyes, wondering bitterly why I let myself acknowledge the full depth of my feelings for him only when I safely knew it could be indulged infrequently. As I wrote in my diary, "If I don't love him, why did I cry so painfully when it came time for him to leave? If I do love him, why has our relationship fluctuated so wildly the last few years? A riddle I long since gave up on. Anyway, it's awful being alone again . . ."

It was so awful that within a few weeks of arriving at Yale, I decided I had to go back into therapy.

IV

In 1957, upon his return to Yale as a faculty member, Duberman finds himself beset by an ulcer, depression, and anxiety about his abilities as a teacher. University scandals of that time involving the discharge of gay faculty members further add to his anxieties:

It was time, I reasoned, to return to therapy. I didn't want (as I wrote in my diary) "to start the pain and upset of analysis all over again," yet felt I had to. At twenty-seven, my career was moving along well but my personal life seemed a shambles. I'd moved away from my friends and lost my lover, had developed an ulcer, felt mostly blue, occasionally manic, never peaceful.

The therapist I chose this time was "Dr. Albert Igen," a professor of psychiatry at the Yale Medical School. I liked him immediately. Low-keyed and compassionate, he refrained from pompous pronouncements and optimistic predictions alike, telling me that for the sake of a "sounder adjustment" we should indeed work to change my sexual orientation, but that there was no guarantee of success. "It will largely depend," he solemnly told me, "on your wish to change. The ultimate rewards will be great, but since the process of change is fraught with frustration and difficulty, you must greatly want that change in order for it to happen." We agreed on three sessions a week, at twenty dollars a session. That was difficult for me to manage financially, even with occasional help from my parents. In asking for that help, I told them I was going into therapy to resolve a few "marginal issues" in my life.

Igen's tentativeness, in happy contrast to Weintraupt's certitude, seemed to me an encouraging sign. Yet the day after I met with Igen, I felt unaccountably depressed. Perhaps I sensed–certainly it was not conscious–that in the guise of self improvement I had in fact inaugurated yet another round of self-sabotage. By that evening my stomach was rumbling away, and on impulse–psychiatry would have said "in resistance to the commitment I had just made to health"–I decided to tour the New Haven bars. As I wrote in my diary, "So I risk my job–I'm sufficiently depressed not to care. If I could stand still and *understand the* depression . . . I'd no doubt be better off. But homosexuality has been a channel–*the* channel–for so long that it's easier to keep running."

When I reported the excursion to Igen, he said he agreed with Weintraupt–though Igen employed a mournful rather than peremptory tone–that change would come only if I proved willing to sit with my "problems," working on them slowly and deliberately in therapy instead of "acting them out." I said that I had tried all that before, with Dr. Weintraupt, and that the strain had proven intolerable. Igen's response was temperate: "You are now older and wiser, better able to withstand the need for instant gratification. Besides, the injunction from your therapist now coincides more exactly with what you feel within. In your healthier moments, you *know* that your sexual compulsions are destructive and should be resisted. But the decision to resist must, of course, be yours."

Perhaps because he didn't press me for an immediate commitment to celibacy, I said I would try, though I wasn't feeling optimistic about my chances on either side of the equation. As I wrote that night in my diary, "The prospects of a lasting homosexual relationship are too slim for me to get much comfort from the possibility; and a satisfying heterosexual relationship is still so remote that I can barely even wish for it. But perhaps either luck in the first area or Dr. Igen in the latter will make one or the other come true. In the meantime, I remain skeptical and unhappy."

I sat still for a whole month. Then Dr. Igen told me he had to have an eye operation and would be out of the office for four or five weeks. I cried a little, possibly with relief, told him I would try to hold the fort but didn't see how I could do that without having the support of continual therapy sessions. He said again, this time with more than a trace of impatience, "That decision is yours."

[On Memorial Day weekend of 1958, Duberman goes to Fire Island where he meets and falls in love with "Billy."] Dr. Igen tried to calm me down. He said the intensity of my reaction, and especially my fear that Billy wouldn't reciprocate my feelings, suggested an archetypal drama only incidentally related to Billy himself. With prodding, I supplied the archetype: my father. A sweet but distant man, he had met my attempts at closeness, as a child, with vague indifference. I would produce that same unhappy outcome with Billy, Igen warned, unless I worked hard to understand and control my impulse to bind him to my side. But this was no time for caution, I protested. Having finally met someone I felt I could care for, didn't it make sense to let my feelings be known and to pursue them? Hadn't I in general been too cautious with my life, working my way methodically through the academic traces, dutifully churning out the required doctoral thesis, quietly following the rules for institutional success?

Perhaps, Igen replied. But I had the cart before the horse. The cure for feelings of professional sterility was not a half-baked leap into emotional turmoil. My current concentration should be on my therapy; until I resolved my conflicts, I could not hope to improve either my professional or my personal life. There was real merit to Igen's argument, as my stormy relationship with Billy would prove. But Igen never saw (or acknowledged) that some fair portion of my conflicts arose from therapeutic assumptions themselves about the pathology of homosexuality, and that it was the cautious climate of the day, rather than the needs of an individual patient, that dictated his automatic suspicion of risk-taking of any kind.

I didn't see any of that either, of course, and in my diary dutifully parroted Igen's wary views: "To make any radical changes in my life without first securing my emotions, would in all likelihood be only exchanging one set of discontents for another." Yet I refused to bow entirely to prudent advice (a rebellious underside would always prove my saving grace). To counteract my feelings of discontent with the world of scholarship, I "daringly" decided not to spend all of my free time converting my doctoral dissertation on Charles Francis Adams into a full-scale biography and to use some of it to explore my long-standing impulse to write a play. In my late teens I had toured with an acting company, and although, at parental urging, I had given up the idea of making the theater my career, its appeal had remained.

I also decided, despite the odds, to pursue the affair with Billy. He was a sweet man. It seems right to fall in love with goodness, so long as one remembers (not easy for those of us socialized to be men) that goodness is not an aphrodisiac, and can desist from blaming the relationship or oneself when comfort displaces passion. That was even harder to manage in the fifties, for the emphasis then was on the inseparability of love and sex, on their happy and perpetual union. After the first few months of absorbing ecstasy, Billy and I lapsed into a reciprocal affection that made me feel peacefully connected–but not particularly turned on.

We both viewed the decline in erotic excitement as a negative judgment on our prospective compatibility and for the next six months tried to figure out whether we could salvage domesticity by sacrificing monogamy. Agreeing that complete fidelity was impossible anyway, since males (we had been taught) were promiscuous "by nature," we tried giving each other a loose rein except when together on weekends. It didn't work. Even though neither of us in fact roamed very far, I couldn't shake the notion that a roving eye signaled cosmic disabilities. Ten months after we'd met, Billy and I threw in the towel.

By winter, I had a second ulcer. Dr. Igen used it to sound his old themes with new urgency. After nearly a year and a half of therapy, he said, it was time for me to take hold. The failure of the affair with Billy should have conclusively demonstrated to me, Igen said, the futility of investing my hopes for sustained intimacy in a homosexual relationship. It was time to look elsewhere, time to close the "escape hatch," confront my underlying anxiety, move toward a heterosexual adjustment.

My assent was less automatic this time around, a rudimentary resistance apparent in the tone I took when pondering Igen's near-ultimatum in an April 1959 diary entry:

> I haven't as yet really resolved in my mind whether I want to make the "grand effort" or, instead, give up the analysis. No small part of my discontent has sprung from the tension which analysis itself has set up. For six years now I've been made ever more aware of the difference between the way I act and the way I *should* act. I've never attempted what possibly could be a satisfactory homosexual adjustment because I've never been sure that I had to settle for that. If I once decided that I was unwilling–perhaps unable–to give up my drives and go through the prolonged agony necessary for a "conversion," then I would be forced to accept my present condition and make the best of it. Once the frame was definitely established, I could work within it toward a reasonable adjustment.

I was still using words like "settle" and "condition," and I quickly went on in the diary to disavow my own rebellious thoughts:

> On the other hand, I recoil from the finality which all this implies. I'm too aware of the inadequacies of homosexual life, of the limited relationships and the emotional constriction, to willingly consign myself to it. And if there are serious difficulties now, how much more intensified will they be in ten years, when my physical attractiveness has faded. Perhaps the situation is literally insoluble.

[Duberman meets a graduate student, "Nancy," who is engaged to someone back home in Toronto] We took to each other immediately. Sharing similar backgrounds–immigrant Jewish fathers who became financially successful; dynamic, native-born mothers who had never been encouraged to use their gifts and had turned querulous–we also had many of the same personality traits. We were ambitious, competitive, obsessive, complaining, and hard-working, and had articulate social charms that concealed far less tidy interiors. With temperaments matching right down to a shared penchant for self-dramatizing humor, Nancy and I were like brother-and-sister clones. Yet we never quite gave up the idea that we might become lovers.

For two years we danced around that possibility. In the back of my mind was Igen's voice, enthusiastically urging me on; in the back of Nancy's was her starchy fiancé's insistence on monogamy. Still, as she told me many years later, after she and her fiancé had long since married, she was "pretty sure" we would have become lovers if I had wanted to. I didn't, but I tried hard to coax the desire into being. We would have a few drinks of an evening in my apartment, turn on music and dance, kiss gently on the lips, and wait expectantly for my body to go into hormonal overdrive–which it never did.

My lack of interest deeply puzzled me. Without doubt Nancy and I were ideally suited, sharing values, open and warm in our affection, comfortable and trusting; we did love each other. It seemed downright unfair–a comment on the malign illogic of the universe–that such entire compatibility would not be blessed with a little usable lust. I tried not to think of friendship–knowing how rare it was–as a consolation prize for those who couldn't manage the main event. But focused as I was on my inadequacy as a lover, it was hard to feel grateful for my talent as a friend.

Dr. Igen kept the focus steady. He encouraged me to speculate about the source of my "unconscious resistance" to physical love with a woman. Though rarely theoretical, he made reference to a possible "breast complex" and asked me if I had reacted violently to being weaned. When I laughed and said I couldn't remember as far back as yesterday's movie, let alone my experiences in the crib, he replied, with a pained expression, that that too was part of the resistance.

Alarmed at how sulky he looked (would he tell me I was hopeless? would he give up on me?), I offered in quick substitution a lengthy speculation about how unlikely it was that a mother as devoted as mine would have weaned me prematurely and thus provoked my rage. His expression lightened a bit, and he took up the theme of my mother's devotion. "Yes," he said, "devotion embedded in control, devotion as a mask for seduction. Is it any wonder you have had difficulty ever since in entrusting yourself to a female? You're chronically angry at women and refuse to get it up for them. To enter a vagina is for you to risk being swallowed alive."

That brought us back to Nancy. I worried aloud about the morality–while working through my "resistance"–of "leading Nancy on." I recognized her own ambivalence about our sleeping together, but didn't that at least partly relate to the confusion she felt at my lack of desire? And wouldn't it be kinder and more honorable simply to tell her that I was sexually attracted to men, not women?

Igen would have none of it. He assured me that the real immorality would be to blurt out the truth about my homosexuality. "That would be a disservice to both of you," he would say. "After all, homosexuality may soon be a thing of the past with you, and to bring it up would be to sabotage any prospect for a different kind of future." Such optimism, as I turned thirty, seemed increasingly fanciful, but I wanted to believe him. After all, I had known other gay men who had married, who had functioned well enough sexually to have children, and who had seemed content. Their strategies for dealing with homosexual urges varied from secret trips to the baths to celibacy (extending, after a while, to their wives). Why let the small matter of lust stand between one and the certified good life?

I eased my conscience about being dishonest with Nancy by periodically throwing out oblique hints. When, for reasons of her own, she turned a deaf ear to them, I occasionally became more explicit and once described in some detail a recent bar pickup in New York. Nancy treated the revelation as an isolated, even bold adventure, and we went on as before.

It wasn't until 1961, as she was preparing to go back to Canada, that I *insisted* she hear the full truth. Years later Nancy recalled in a letter to me how *"stunned"* she had been at the news: "I remember quite literally not sleeping for the next two nights, and being in a state of absolute internal tumult. It was all beyond my experience–and the more so because my emotions were engaged." She mulled over the possibility of staying on in New Haven, making me into something like a project, helping me to "break through" into heterosexuality. Doubtless Dr. Igen and his colleagues would have applauded her impulse; to this day the popular cure-all for homosexuality is (for gay men) "the love of a good woman" and (for lesbians) "a good fuck." But Nancy had sounder instincts and headed home to safer shores.

[In 1961, Duberman first develops hepatitis and then another illness] Painful sores appeared on my penis, so painful I nervously recalled biblical plagues and punishments. No, the doctor said, nothing so apocalyptic: "You have herpes simplex, a frequent aftermath of hepatitis. The sores will subside, but never disappear."

"Never?!"

"Once you contract the virus, you always have it in your system. But you can go for long periods of time without its being active."

In those pre-acyclovir years, no satisfactory treatment existed for herpes; one tried everything, including prayer. I began what would turn into a sixteen-month pilgrimage to dermatologists' offices in search of relief–after a while, in search just of hope. One dermatologist recommended constant "warm soaks," and for a month–until superseded by a later nostrum–I wandered the apartment with my penis submerged in a glass of warm water. I even got adept at talking on the phone, lips chattering away about my latest Lowell research [Duberman was writing James Russell Lowell's biography] or departmental crisis, eyes fixed lugubriously on my flaccid, scab-flecked organ floating senselessly in its liquid bath.

It was now useless with a vengeance. Igen suggested that the affliction contained a message we needed to decode and an opportunity we needed to seize. The message, as we worked it out, had to do–surprise!– with my unconscious. Having despaired of my ability consciously to control my sexual acting out with men, I had let my unconscious–in touch with my deep, continuing desire for a heterosexual adjustment–take over. Wondrously intricate in its workings, my unconscious had come up with a brilliant solution. It had created all at once an unarguable physical obstacle to sexual activity, a set of real physical symptoms on which I could focus some of my generalized anxiety, and an arresting symbolic visualization of my inner state–the sick penis as a representation of my underlying sense of worthlessness. It was now my job to carry this impressive subterranean achievement onto a conscious level, to accept and incorporate its insights as rational guides to behavior. If I succeeded in doing that, Igen triumphantly predicted, I would no longer have to hold on to the viral infection as a safeguard against future backsliding.

While I was still in the throes of this bewildering set of symptoms and injunctions, my biography of Charles Francis Adams was published to a fine set of notices, including the front page of *The New York Times Book Review*. Soon after came the announcement that the book had won the Bancroft Prize. And soon after that came an offer from Princeton for me to join its history department, with a raise in both pay and rank over what I had at Yale. The damage herpes had done to my ego seemed all but repaired. Igen expressed regret that I would leave therapy just when I was making "great strides" and, equating enforced celibacy with inner conversion, seemed "on the verge of a cure." But he agreed that the Princeton offer was too good to turn down. He wished me all the best and urged me to "stay in touch."

Becoming Gay:
A Personal Odyssey

Richard A. Isay, MD

We seek other conditions because we know not how to enjoy our own;
and to go outside Of ourselves for want of knowing what it is like inside
Of us.

–Montaigne

In Yale's psychiatry department during the 1960s, most of us studying to
become psychiatrists believed that psychoanalysis was the optimal therapy for
emotional disorders. The analyst, with his esoteric technique that included a
couch, free association, and four or five sessions a week over at least that many
years, appeared to have greater access to the hidden recesses of his own mind,
as well as to the mind of others, than did the psychiatrist in his face-to-face,
once or twice-weekly therapy. Psychoanalysis also offered an all-encompass-
ing theory of mental functioning and human development, and reading Freud
was not only intellectually engaging but great fun. The majority of psychiatric
residents at that time wanted to be analyzed; many of us hoped to become analysts.

I had wanted to be a psychoanalyst since my third year at Haverford College. In a course on nineteenth-century philosophy I had read Schopenhauer
and Nietzsche, whose views about irrational sources of human behavior and

Richard A. Isay is Clinical Professor of Psychiatry, Weill Medical College of Cor-
nell University and on the faculty of the Columbia University Center for Psychoanalytic Training and Research.

[Haworth co-indexing entry note]: "Becoming Gay: A Personal Odyssey." Isay, Richard A. Co-published
simultaneously in *Journal of Gay & Lesbian Psychotherapy* (The Haworth Medical Press, an imprint of The
Haworth Press, Inc.) Vol. 5, No. 3/4, 2001, pp. 51-67; and: *Sexual Conversion Therapy: Ethical, Clinical and
Research Perspectives* (ed: Ariel Shidlo, Michael Schroeder, and Jack Drescher) The Haworth Medical Press,
an imprint of The Haworth Press, Inc., 2001, pp. 51-67.

the unconscious mind intrigued me. Jung's speculative thinking about myths, archetypes, and archetypal images provided a bridge between my interest in philosophy and a growing fascination with academic psychology. I had no idea that my burgeoning interest in the mind was due to distress and confusion over a longstanding attraction to other boys.

In my freshman year I had fallen in love with one of my classmates. I first saw Bob on the train returning to college from Thanksgiving vacation. He had a slender, well-proportioned, athletic body, dark hair, which he wore in a neat brush cut, soft but intelligent brown eyes, and a warm, engaging smile. I thought he was incredibly handsome. I admired how comfortable he was with our classmates and how much they, in turn, appeared to want him to like them. Although too shy to speak to him on the train, I noted his every move and developed a crush and the determination to get to know him. We lived near each other in the same dormitory, and with a studied nonchalance that belied my excitement I'd drop over to his room to chat. We gradually became friends and decided to live together the following year. I moved into the suite he was sharing with two roommates.

In my sophomore year a recent graduate of Harvard's clinical psychology program had joined Haverford's faculty to teach psychology. He was a demanding and dynamic teacher, interested in psychoanalytic theory and the contributions psychoanalysis had made to understanding human motivation and behavior. In his course on personality we read Freud's views on homosexuality as a perversion, and I became convinced that I was sick. But from what I learned the next semester about adolescence in his course on human development, I comforted myself with the knowledge that some attraction to other boys was natural and that my infatuation with Bob was a passing phase that would soon be replaced by an equally passionate interest in girls.

Since I was never attracted to girls, I dated infrequently. My evenings and weekends were spent studying, often simply to avoid the appearance of having time on my hands. My roommates were all diligent students. Bob was pre-med and worked hard, although his considerable academic achievements often appeared effortless. Another roommate, Jack, was the college German scholar, who immersed himself in German literature in addition to his premedical studies. Their dedication to academic pursuits, along with my own, usually made it unnecessary for me to date except on rare occasions such as the annual college dance, when I felt social pressure to do so.

I looked forward to the time that Bob and I spent alone and was jealous when he was with other friends, particularly his girlfriend. I fantasized about spending the rest of my life with him, longed to have unlimited access to him and the time and freedom to touch and be close to him forever. I knew that I had fallen in love, but I believed it was due to his being a kind and thoughtful person. The idea that my desire was the passionate expression of a sexual orientation never crossed my mind. Although Bob and I engaged in casual sexual play, I did not label myself "homosexual." I did view my attraction to him as a serious neurotic problem since I was uncertain that I fell into the category of those "normal" adolescents who simply had occasional thoughts about other boys.

Midway in my third year of college I was concerned enough about my attachment to Bob to attempt to speak about it with my psychology professor. On the way to his office I recalled his response to a student who had asked him how to distinguish between an eighteen- or nineteen-year-old who had normal homosexual thoughts from someone who was actually homosexual. "You might worry," he had said, "if you see a soldier in uniform, he looks attractive, and you wonder what his body looks like." By the time I had arrived at the office door, convinced that he would think I was homosexual even though I was unable to, I decided not to mention being in love and, instead, spoke with him about my career indecision. I thought I detected some incredulity when he asked me if anything else was troubling me, and I uncomfortably responded, "No."

In fact, I was concerned about my future career plans. By the second semester of that junior year I had decided to go to graduate school in clinical psychology in order to become a psychoanalyst, a decision that I knew was partly motivated by concern over my own emotional distress and the belief that I could benefit from treatment. But in the spring of that year, as president of the Haverford-Bryn Mawr Psychology Club, I had the opportunity to spend time with the famous psychoanalyst Erich Fromm, who had been invited to lecture at the college. He was accompanied by his blond and attractive second wife, who seemed quite a bit younger than he. I was impressed by how adoring they were of each other, and though it was clear he would have preferred being alone with his new wife, I took every opportunity to talk with him about the future direction of my career. Fromm had studied sociology and political science before psychoanalysis, but he advised me to go to medical school and become a psychiatrist before receiving psychoanalytic training, assuring me that psychiatry offered more career opportunities and financial security than psychology did at the time.

By the end of my junior year I had decided to follow his advice, and I began to take the necessary and arduous premedical courses the following year. Neither my senior year of college, in which I began my premedical studies, the postgraduate year in which I completed them, nor my first two years of medical school studying the preclinical sciences held much academic interest. These courses, however, kept me preoccupied and depressed. I was both too busy to date women and too distressed to be aware of my homosexual desire.

Bob told me in the spring of our last year of college that he planned to marry immediately after graduation. Jealous and angry, I tearfully opposed his marriage and told him so. He listened patiently, but seemed relieved that I would be traveling during the summer and unable to attend his wedding. When I visited him on occasional weekends the following years in Boston, where he was in medical school, I was consumed by anguish and jealousy whenever he and his wife would retire to their bedroom. Depression over my separation from him contributed to my lack of interest in sex during this period.

I was aware that I had homosexual masturbation fantasies and was occasionally conscious of longing for sexual contact with men, but I continued to believe that my desires were symptoms of emotional difficulties that could eventually be cured. I had read enough psychoanalysis to be convinced, as analysts then believed, that if I was not having sex, I was not really homosexual. Also, at the time I was convinced that in order to be accepted for training as a psychiatrist or as a psychoanalyst I would have to be heterosexual, so in my second year of medical school I set out with determination to date women.

The summer before my third year I met my future wife. We went out several times that summer while I was in New York City on a fellowship and she was home from college. I thought it was a sign of the severity of my emotional problems that I was not attracted to women, and my lack of passion made me more eager than ever to begin treatment. With the help of an analyst, and providing I did not give in to my homosexual impulses, I believed that I would be able to put such feelings out of my mind and eventually be able to marry.

I did not contact her for another three years. Although exhaustion during my internship year in Cleveland had extinguished most of my social inclinations and much of my sexual desire, I did notice my attraction to some of the men I shared on-call rooms with. I became eager to start treatment the following year to rid myself of these unwanted impulses.

Two months after beginning my training in psychiatry at Yale, I started to look for an analyst. I spoke with two. Both were certified to analyze candidates in psychoanalytic training, so I assumed that they would be knowledgeable and clinically proficient. The first was the chairman of the Education Committee of the Western New England Institute for Psychoanalysis in New Haven. When I called to speak with him, his secretary told me that I could make an appointment only by writing and describing the nature of the difficulties for which I felt I needed to be treated. Since he was educational director of the institute, I thought he would be the best analyst. I should take note, I believed, of his request to put my problems in writing, since this must have important technical significance. Several years later he told me that he was somewhat phobic and avoided speaking on the telephone except when doing so was unavoidable.

During the consultation he asked me about my sexual experiences with girls. I had no difficulty telling him that I had none since he, overweight, quite bald, and shy, gave the impression that he was asexual. However, even he seemed a bit surprised by my sexual inexperience and inactivity.

I told him about getting turned on by wrestling with my friend Lou in his attic on weekends in high school and the mild sexual activity at college with Bob, but I did not think to tell him I had been in love, since he seemed to be interested only in my sexual behavior and not in my longing for love from a man. Nor did he inquire about my homosexual masturbation fantasies. He was reassured by my relative lack of homosexual experience and by the fact that I was once again trying to date. At that time I shared his conviction that homosexuality was simply a matter of sex, not of love, and that if I did not "act out" my desire then I was emotionally disturbed, but not homosexual, and could become heterosexual.

I liked this man because of his lack of pretension and his emotional responsiveness. I felt strangely comforted by his obvious eccentricities. I was flattered that he offered to take me on as a patient, but he could see me only once a week until he had more time available to begin an analysis the following year. Believing I could be "cured" only if I saw someone daily, I decided to look for another analyst.

Ruben Samuels was by reputation a "nice guy." He was in his mid-fifties and was also designated by the American Psychoanalytic Association to train future analysts. He seemed to be kind, intelligent, and patient, although somewhat depressed. He was encouraged that I had not had sex with a man since college and was clearly enthusiastic about my continuing to date. He seemed very "normal." I had even heard that he swam regularly at the Jewish community center, which, since I had never been athletic, gave me an added sense that, unlike myself, he was a thoroughly heterosexual person. Although his apparent normality made me feel uneasy, I decided to start analysis as soon as he had an opening, which would be a few months from our first consultation. I had found an analyst like the father I would have wanted.

My father had died suddenly of a myocardial infarction three days after my twelfth birthday. He had left college during his first year to work, and, although warmer and certainly kinder than my mother, he also lacked her education and cultural interests. His friends seemed, like him, to be inclined to sports and little interested in intellectual pursuits. I was shy, withdrawn, awkward, and unathletic. I've always believed that I disappointed him by not being masculine enough.

My analyst appeared to be kind and masculine like my father, but he also had the intellectual curiosity and culture that my father had seemed to lack. And since we shared an enthusiasm for psychoanalysis, I believed I had a chance to redo the relationship with my father.

Although I was a good psychiatry resident and enjoyed my work, I felt lonely, depressed, and, at times, desperate. I thought that my despair was the result of an inability to express my inhibited heterosexuality; I never imagined that it could be the result of the denial and suppression of my homosexuality. I had recognized by then how strong my homosexual feelings were and, most likely, knew unconsciously the futility of attempting to arouse the "blighted germs" of my purported heterosexuality; however, since I thought of myself as being emotionally disturbed and not gay, I had never contemplated finding sexual and emotional gratification with another man.

I had liked my future wife from the time we met. I knew she had the qualities of character and intelligence of someone I could marry. But I had not contacted her until one month before my consultation with Dr. Samuels. I desperately wanted to please him and tried to do so by anticipating his wish that I give up my homosexual desire by dating and having sex with girls.

I had been waiting for about eight years to begin treatment; the four months between consulting with my future analyst and starting the analysis felt endless. On the day we finally began, Dr. Samuels explained the basic rules of saying whatever came to my mind. I lay down on the couch and wept about my loneliness and inability to experience any passion. After a few days, we decided that analysis six times a week rather than the usual four or five seemed indicated because of the severity of my heterosexual inhibition and considerable unhappiness.

Like all analysts at the time, he advocated and promoted my own conviction that sexual attraction to men was a serious emotional affliction. He implied that by becoming aware of the childhood fear of my father's rage over my closeness to my mother I would become less frightened of the mortal consequences of my heterosexual desire, heterosexuality would flower, and homosexual desire would subside.

In the second year of analysis I had sex with a woman for the first time, but I was persistently anxious about losing my erection, which happened with discomforting frequency. Sex was neither passionate nor fun. In that same year, for a brief time, I developed a distressing symptom of genital anesthesia, a symptom that Dr. Samuels interpreted as a symbolic autocastration that expressed my anxiety about becoming increasingly heterosexual. His interpretation of the childhood terror of my father's retaliation had little effect on my impotence. Only after I had completed analysis did I understand that the genital numbness had been another way of trying to please my analyst, since it kept me from masturbating and having the homosexual fantasies that were tellingly present whenever I did.

In my third year of analysis my future wife and I became engaged. My analyst, who had never called me by name in our sessions because he felt it would interfere with the perception of his neutrality, enthusiastically congratulated me. And although he was on vacation at the time, he sent a warm telegram to the synagogue on the occasion of our marriage the following summer.

During the early years, frequent impotence became persistent whenever Ruben went on vacation, a symptom that he interpreted again and again as being caused by fear of my heterosexuality and the repressed anxiety, grief, and anger over the untimely death of my father at the onset of my adolescence. It was not until I had finished analysis that I understood that what episodic heterosexual behavior I had been capable of had been motivated by my desire to please my analyst, and when he went on vacation my heterosexuality did as well.

The denial of my homosexuality had always been strong, and now the daily contact with my analyst, who usually implicitly but sometimes explicitly conveyed his view that I was a neurotically inhibited heterosexual, provided me with little opportunity to consider the idea that I was homosexual.

Furthermore, my desire to be a psychoanalyst was contributing to the denial of my homosexuality. Analysts assumed that the same early trauma that caused one to become homosexual produced such severe personality defects that analysts who themselves were homosexual would be unable to sustain the emotional constraint, neutrality, attentiveness, and empathy that enable one to do competent therapy. Therefore, persons who were actively homosexual were not accepted for training at psychoanalytic institutes affiliated with the American Psychoanalytic Association. Since I was making an effort to rid myself of homosexual fantasies and to disinhibit my heterosexuality, I believed I could be accepted and decided to apply for psychoanalytic training.

Three senior analysts interviewed me. Although I was cautiously truthful about my sexual history, the Education Committee undoubtedly saw my eagerness to spend one hour every day labeling myself neurotic as a sign of emotional health. Furthermore, it seemed impossible for psychoanalytic educators, as it had been for my analyst, to reconcile the reputation I had as a psychiatry resident who had done good clinical work with patients with the idea that I could be homosexual. I did not look or act like all homosexuals were assumed to appear or behave–effeminate, odd, or in some other way unconventional. It was for these reasons, I believe, and because I was not "acting out" my sexual fantasies, that the Education Committee did not consider me to be homosexual and I was accepted for training.

I continued my analysis with Dr. Samuels. My self-image and self-esteem did improve somewhat as a result of the recollection of troublesome aspects of my childhood that had been repressed. My depression, however, did not improve, due to the difficulty I now experienced having any sexual feelings or impulses whatsoever. I also had a problem thinking clearly around my analyst. He believed all these symptoms were caused by anxiety about showing him my masculine aggressiveness because I feared him as I had feared my father. But the aggressiveness I was anxious about had nothing to do with masculinity, as he had suggested; it was caused by a need to inhibit my mounting anger with him. I was devoting most of my psychic energy to repressing my sexuality and anger and was consequently becoming more depressed. I was getting worse, not better.

I was the middle of three children, placed between an athletically inclined older brother, who I felt was preferred by both my parents, and a sister three years younger who was clearly adored because of her cute, winning ways. I was awkward, shy, and overweight, and when my sister was born, I believed, as do many children, that my parents were eager to have her so they could get rid of me. She was the object of much attention, and the more attention she got, the more obstreperous I became.

One of the early memories recollected in my analysis was from soon after my sister's birth, when, feeling neglected by my mother, I refused to leave her to go to bed. Frustrated, she tied me with rope to the mattress and locked my door. Out of terror and fury I struggled to get out of bed, pulling the mattress on top of me, falling asleep exhausted, trying to find air.

Neither of my parents was affectionate, either with each other or with their children. I grew up believing both that expressions of affection were unnatural and that sexual excitement was inappropriate. My father was chronically unhappy and depressed. He often spent entire weekends in bed; we saw little of him and our care was left to my mother. Although she was more tolerant of my lack of athletic prowess and of my aesthetic interests than he, my mother was also swifter to anger. She had felt emotionally deprived by her own parents, particularly by her domineering mother, and she had little patience for the emotional needs of her children. She demanded obedience, and punishment was swift and severe.

Like many homosexual boys, I felt I had been a disappointment to my father. I went to camp to please him, starting at age seven, until the summer after his death, when, at age twelve, relieved, I did not have to return.

The last three years had been particularly difficult. I was then at an athletic camp; we went relentlessly every day from softball to tennis and, with terror, once a week, to boxing. I did enjoy swimming, which was a respite from the demands to compete athletically because I could float for long periods of time. I also enjoyed the changing room and showers, where I watched other boys with a curiosity and enthusiasm that was lacking at other times in my day.

It was a month after returning home from camp and a few days after receiving a report from the director that my father asked me to go for a ride with him and a friend. I was excited to be with him, seated in the front seat between him and an obviously powerfully built man. He asked me to feel his friend's large muscular arms. "That," he said, "is how I want you to look." I was deeply embarrassed. I was sure his heart had been chilled by the report that I was uncoordinated, immature, and the "outstanding homesick boy of the season." He died six months later, at age forty-five, of a heart attack.

Soon after his death my mother began to comment about my being over-weight, awkward, too shy, and unathletic. I imagine she feared that a sensitive, shy adolescent who shunned competitive sports and lacked a masculine pres-ence might become homosexual. She asked the family pediatrician to talk to me about sex. After a thorough physical exam, he lectured me about the rela-tionship between healthy exercise and a clean mind. He assured me that exer-cise would also make me look "more like a boy." He suggested that I do situps and cautioned me about masturbating, which I had not yet attempted, but which, soon thereafter, I successfully tried.

My masturbation must have come to my mother's attention, since a friend of my father's came over to our house one evening soon after I had discovered how to do it to tell me not to and to warn that it could interfere with my liking girls. While not deterring me, these talks did make me wary of having any erotic thoughts. They also contributed to my growing conviction that sexual excitement was not only inappropriate but bad and harmful. While in analysis I grew to believe that my parents' inability to express affection and to convey a sense of their own sexuality, along with the discouragement of my sexuality as an adolescent, had all contributed to the inhibition of my adult heterosexual de-sire. After my analysis, I understood that my belief that all sex was bad helped to explain why I had persistently denied my homosexuality and why I thought it to be a sickness.

Recollection of childhood memories, some of which had been repressed, was helpful in improving my sense of selfworth, but my analyst's conviction that homosexual impulses were simply a defense against my latent heterosexu-ality made me feel more defective because I could no longer experience any passion. Although increasingly hopeless, I continued to obey his implicit ad-monitions not to "act out" homosexual impulses, which we both understood could cause my dismissal from the psychoanalytic training program or, at least, an interruption until such behavior ceased.

Analysts at most institutes were required to report their patients' progress to the Education Committee in order for a candidate to progress to didactic courses and to treat patients under supervision. The implicit power held by one's training analyst, no matter how well intentioned or protective of confi-dentiality he was, could at times inhibit any analysand's behavior, thoughts, and fantasies. Because I did trust my analyst's discretion and believed that the reporting requirements at my institute were minimal and would not require vi-olations of confidentiality, I was not conscious of concerns that my behavior or homosexual impulses would hinder the progression of my career. Neverthe-less, unconscious fear of being reported undoubtedly added to the difficulties I continued to have in acknowledging to myself that I was homosexual.

In the fall of 1971 my analyst raised the question of terminating treatment. I had been seeing him for nearly ten years and, for seven of these years, six times a week; for three years, five times weekly. He felt we had done as much work as possible.

I was now rarely functioning sexually, and when I did it was with great effort. I had rationalized that maturity and mental health demanded the sublimation of sexual excitement in work and in responsibility for the welfare of others. I was also relieved by the idea of stopping. It meant that I had my analyst's approval and would soon graduate from the institute, the first of my class of candidates to do so. The date my analyst and I had set for the actual termination was about eight months from that time, which gave us an opportunity to deal with old conflicts and transference issues that would manifest themselves in the face of terminating.

On at least two occasions during that last year I browsed gay pornography in New Haven bookstores. My analyst and I concurred that I was attempting to sabotage my career as well as my marriage and that this behavior was motivated by anger at him for stopping treatment. He reminded me that I had felt both abandoned and relieved when my father had died, believing that these old feelings were being revived in the transference.

His observations were partly correct. However, neither of us then understood that the prospect of terminating and of not having to comply in the future with his expectations of heterosexuality was enabling me to feel somewhat more comfortable expressing my homosexual desire and inclinations.

When I finished my analysis, I was in my mid-thirties and had a wife and two children, all of whom I loved. By then I had stopped having sex because I no longer felt a need to please my analyst by continuing to try. My unsuccessful efforts had caused me more anguish than pleasure, so I was relieved. But I was a caring husband and father, felt guilty about depriving my wife of sex, and viewed my lack of heterosexual passion as a serious deficiency.

Childhood rivalries with my brother and sister, the longing for the love of both my parents, and the pain and anger I experienced from feeling unappreciated by them no longer affected my current relationships as they had before my analysis. I was now better equipped to recognize these old feelings when they reemerged with my wife, children, colleagues, patients, and friends. I had discovered new ways of dealing with them that were no longer so self-defeating, spiteful, or defensive. But because of my analyst's heterosexual bias, I was further from understanding at the end of analysis than at the start that my lack of heterosexual desire was due to my being homosexual.

An analyst or therapist who sees his patient four or five or, as in my case, six times a week induces a passivity that encourages in most an acquiescence, compliance, and responsiveness to his views no matter how indirectly suggestions are made or how careful he is to attempt to remain neutral. I had been told repeatedly that my homosexual impulses were but ways of inhibiting my heterosexuality and, since I wanted to believe it, had unquestioningly accepted my analyst's perception that I was an impaired heterosexual.

Shortly after we stopped, I began to experience and express more anger and to think about why I had had trouble with these emotions during my treatment. The problem had been caused partly by the difficulty my analyst had had allowing me to be angry with him. In my consultation he had set forth the rule that I was not to consider him late until he was more than five minutes late. Our hours frequently did not start on time, but if he was ten minutes late and I complained, he would wonder why I was so angry since, according to our agreement, he was only five minutes late. If he was less than five minutes late and I complained, then he insisted I must be displacing my anger about someone or something else onto him since he was not to be considered late at all until after five minutes. His logic consistently enraged me, but I learned to suppress my anger, understanding that he did not like confrontation and had difficulty being seen as flawed.

After terminating the analysis, I also thought about the death of my father, recalling that at my birthday dinner I had attempted to make a declaration of rights for twelve-year olds, which included the right to smoke. He disagreed and I argued and, being unable to impose my will, furiously left the table. His sudden death a few days later, along with my mother's physical punishments, had convinced me that disagreement with authority in the pursuit of my own conviction would always have disastrous consequences–another reason I had a problem expressing anger while I was in treatment.

It was only three or four months after stopping analysis that I again began to have vivid homosexual fantasies, impulses, and dreams. It was then I recognized that I had been denying and repressing homosexual feelings because I had longed for my analyst's approval and that one way to please him had been to comply with his conviction that I was not homosexual. I knew my need for his approval had been an unanalyzed aspect of the transference, inadvertently used by him in his attempt to make me heterosexual.

Finished with my analysis, I no longer felt passive and compliant and was more comfortable with my anger. I also had less need for social approbation, having learned in my analysis how this need had been caused by feeling unloved as a child. Furthermore, the love I got from my wife and children, along with my professional success, had enhanced my self confidence.

Six months after completing treatment, while in New York at the fall meeting of the American Psychoanalytic Association, I went to a gay pornographic movie. Within a few minutes, because of the intensity of my sexual feelings, I realized that, in fact, I was homosexual. For the first time, because my sexual feelings and impulses were so clear and powerful, I did not believe I was sick. I experienced a sense of relief and exhilaration. I knew that homosexuality was the passion I had believed myself incapable of ever experiencing.

For the next weeks elation alternated with intense and utter despair. I was devoted to my wife and two children and was nearing completion of training in a profession that was prejudiced against and intolerant of homosexuals. I was excited by the prospect of expressing my sexual passion, but I could not conceive how the confines of my life would ever permit this.

Closeted because of my marriage and my profession and terrified of being discovered, I was able to express my sexuality only in anonymous encounters. One convenient place to have sex was a rest stop on the Connecticut Thruway near New Haven. On one occasion in late 1974, a man who had been acting and responding sexually identified himself as an undercover police officer. He informed me that I was under arrest for lewd conduct in a public accommodation. I was, of course, terrified, envisioning the loss of my family and the destruction of my career. Between the rest room and his patrol car, just as he was about to handcuff me, I talked him out of taking me to the station by forswearing returning to the rest stop, which at that moment seemed both prudent and the last thing I would ever want to do again.

It was customary for the New Haven Register to print the names of those who had been charged with criminal offenses, and I had always taken special note of those booked on "morals" charges. I realized I had placed myself in a situation that had endangered me. I also understood that I must be feeling guilty about my sexuality to have done so and that it had been fear of being discovered that made anonymous encounters the only available way I could have sex. I knew that I would have to find ways to express my sexual desire that would put me in less danger and be more fulfilling. The alternative of not expressing it at all and once again labeling myself as "sick" was no longer possible. My near arrest had shocked me into a pellucid understanding of the practical and psychological dangers inherent in remaining closeted.

Emboldened by the American Psychiatric Association's 1973 decision to remove homosexuality from its Diagnostic and Statistical Manual, I began to think about the antihomosexual bias of psychoanalysis and the adverse ways the view that homosexuals were perverted and should be cured of their illness contributed to the negative image gay men and lesbians have of themselves. I recognized that this bias, which I and my analyst shared, had caused neither of us to question at any time during nearly ten years of treatment why I was suppressing my homosexuality and why I was not permitting myself to have sexual contact with men.

I did not write about these issues for another decade because I was interested in professional advancement, my colleagues' approval, and developing a private practice. Being part of an orthodox Freudian psychoanalytic group, although one more tolerant of divergent views than many other analytic societies, I knew I would be considered too inexperienced to have a valuable opinion about any controversial theoretical or clinical issue. Any such views would simply have been dismissed and would have raised questions about my own sexual orientation.

Over the next few years I wrote and published articles on traditional analytic subjects and became active in the psychoanalytic institute and society. I was appointed to the institute's faculty and Board of Trustees, in 1978 was elected president of the society, and the next year was appointed to important committees of both the American Psychoanalytic and International Psychoanalytical associations.

Feeling isolated by my career and being married and still haunted by the memory of nearly having been arrested, I felt it was essential for my emotional health to share my life as a homosexual with others who could be affirming of my sexual orientation. I had no friends or colleagues with whom I felt comfortable talking about my experiences. I could not speak with my analyst, who would believe I was "acting out" my anxiety and anger and recommend that I reenter analysis. Nor was I yet prepared to talk with my wife.

In 1978 I cautiously began to cruise in New Haven. On one occasion I met a younger, married member of Yale's psychiatry department who, calling himself "bisexual," informed me that there were several other psychiatrists that he knew personally who were married and either gay or bisexual. They met periodically for lunch to provide support for one another, and I immediately made myself known to each of them.

All of these colleagues were respected professionals; two were also members of the psychoanalytic society. Like myself, they were living double lives and having sexual encounters that at one time or another had placed them in physical danger or legal jeopardy. By then I was clearly aware of the role that my childhood, society's prejudice, and my own analysis had played in causing me to deny my homosexuality. I knew that my view that homosexuality was a sickness had been one manifestation of my self-hatred. I recognized that my readiness to "change" and my willingness to submit to a treatment aimed at doing so had also been symptoms of my injured selfesteem. I was, therefore, distressed by how fearful each of us was of being discovered, and I was troubled by the deception we were engaged in to sustain our professional and personal lives.

I was particularly distressed by the effect that my secretiveness was having on my clinical work. By attempting to protect myself from patients' curiosity and scrutiny out of fear that my homosexuality would be exposed, I was never responsive to questions about my personal life. I had, of course, rationalized my need for anonymity as serving my patients' need for an ambiguous object on whom they could project their own fantasies. But my rigidity in this regard was often unnecessarily depriving and sometimes hindered their treatment. I recognized that my energy was being diverted in the clinical situation from self-reflection to self-protection and that fear of being discovered was often interfering with my capacity for empathic response and spontaneity when it was clinically appropriate. The need to hide my sexual orientation was gradually eroding my sense of personal integrity and thereby compromising the honesty that is necessary to sustain the therapeutic endeavor and that contributes to its effectiveness. I became determined to be more "out" as a gay man.

I knew that to be more self-affirming it would be necessary to find gay friends who were open and more comfortable with their sexual orientation than those I had met in New Haven. I had my first opportunity to come out to an openly gay man in 1979, when I met Larry Kramer at a party given by his former therapist and his wife. I had recently read his novel, Faggots, found it caustic and honest, and arranged to meet him at his apartment the next day. When I told him I was gay, Larry attacked me for being closeted and in a profession that had "fucked him up." He told me that the reason I was still closeted was that I was afraid I would lose my patients. He also said I should get divorced. I knew he was partly correct: I was concerned about losing patients. But I did not want a divorce and was concerned about the effect coming out would have on my marriage.

Larry's anger spewed out relentlessly. At the time, of course, I did not know that he would make continued creative use of this anger in his writing and, a few years later, in starting two important organizations, Gay Men's Health Crisis (GMHC) and Act Up. I wondered only whether all future experiences of coming out would make people so angry and be so painful. But I liked his honesty and admired his incisive intelligence. I have felt bonded to him over the years, not only because of my unabashed, if somewhat wary, admiration but because my analyst, Larry told me, had been his therapist when he was a Yale undergraduate.

A few weeks later, while in New York attending professional meetings, I went to a bar where I met a tall, slender man with beautiful auburn hair and striking brown and olive-green eyes. He was bright and inquisitive, and his capacity for self reflection and understanding was immediately evident. Aside from his perceptiveness and sense of humor, Gordon was affectionate, emotionally expressive, candid, and utterly without artifice. Since he was many years younger than I and we came from very different backgrounds, I thought I had met only an intelligent friend with whom I could also have enjoyable sexual encounters. Over the following year I found our differences interesting and that they enhanced the relationship. I was surprised when I discovered that our mutual attachment had deepened and I had fallen in love.

Not long after meeting Gordon, I read a letter in The New York Times from Frank Rundle, who had identified himself as president of the Association of Gay Psychiatrists. I called Frank and made plans to speak with him and the president elect of the association, David Kessler, at the forthcoming meetings of the American Psychiatric Association in San Francisco in May 1980.

Frank and David were the first openly gay mental health professionals with whom I had an opportunity to speak. We shared convictions about the mental health benefits of being out and the need for social and political change within and outside of psychiatry. Their nonjudgmental attitude, understanding, and concern about my difficult social and professional situations were in striking contrast to the attitudes of the closeted psychiatrists and analysts I knew in New Haven, who seemed to view my need to be more open as recklessly endangering my career and marriage and also to be concerned about their exposure were I to become more out.

In 1980, my wife joined me at the psychiatry meetings in San Francisco, where I told her that I was homosexual. Although I did not want a divorce, since I was devoted to her and our sons, then ten and fourteen, it was no longer possible for me to hide my sexual orientation. I believed at the time that it would be possible to be out, when honesty and integrity demanded, and to maintain a viable marriage.

I told her everything I believed she should know about my past and current life, including my relationship with Gordon, that might help her decide about the future direction of her own life and, specifically, whether she wanted to remain in our marriage. My wife was initially relieved that she had not been responsible for my sexual unresponsiveness and appeared to understand both that I needed to express my sexuality and that I loved her and our boys. However, over the next months she made it clear that she wanted me to keep my homosexuality secret to maintain the privacy of the family. We cared a lot about each other and hoped to be able to maintain the relationship, but I feared that her need for secrecy and my need to make my sexual orientation a more positive and better integrated aspect of my self would eventually cause conflict and discord.

Over the next few years, Gordon was often angry about my desire to remain with my family, but he remained respectful of my feelings, agreeing to keep our times together constant each week and careful not to intrude on my life at home. His willingness to sacrifice his own needs for mine meant a great deal, and his thoughtfulness enabled my marriage to continue with reasonable comfort for a few more years.

My family and I moved from New Haven to New York in 1981, after I had spent a year commuting to begin a practice in New York. I started to see many gay men, sent to me by straight colleagues who did not know I was gay. By that time I was responding honestly to inquiries about my sexual orientation, all of which were made by gay patients. My straight patients assumed I was heterosexual because I wore a wedding band, and there were then no known homosexual analysts. My gay patients, generally relieved and pleased that I was also gay, told friends and colleagues. I increasingly got more self referred patients, particularly those who were mental health workers themselves, and my sexual orientation gradually became known.

Since I was chairperson of the American Psychoanalytic Association's Program Committee and secretary of the International Psychoanalytical Association's Program Committee, I now felt I was in a better professional position to raise questions and share what I was learning about the clinical treatment and development of gay men, which had, of course, been importantly shaped by my own experience. I was also in a better personal position to do so since I was out to my wife. For the December 1983 meeting of the American Psychoanalytic Association, I organized and chaired a panel on male homosexuality where I challenged the view of homosexuality as perversion and spoke about some of the men I had seen whose previous analysts had caused psychological damage by attempting to change their sexual orientation. Before that meeting I had had referrals from heterosexual colleagues; afterward, the referrals almost completely ceased. The change in attitude was caused both by colleagues becoming more attentive to rumors about my homosexuality and by my harsh criticism of traditional psychoanalytic theory and practice.

In 1986 I decided to tell my former analyst that I was gay. We had become friendly after I finished my training and occasionally had family dinners and celebrated significant family events together. In spite of my anger at him for not helping me to accept my homosexuality, I liked him, and had become fond of his family and felt that he had helped me in my analysis in other important ways.

I told Ruben about my relationship with Gordon, my increasing need to be out within the gay community, and being more withdrawn and less available to my wife. He looked distressed but had little to say except that he hoped I would be able to live my life in a way that was satisfactory. Our meeting was more perfunctory than I had wished, and sensing his discomfort, I said that I would like to speak with him further and perhaps he could call me whenever he had the time to do so. The call was not forthcoming. I wrote to him, wanting to heal the rift that I felt had been caused by my revelation, mentioned that my life was complex and difficult but challenging and happy and that I was, for the time being, content. He never responded to my letter. I called to ask that he give me a call so we could get together when he was in New York City, but he never did. At its end this relationship recapitulated the rejection I had experienced with my father.

My wife and I had made the decision not to tell the boys about my homosexuality until they seemed developmentally prepared to deal with it. We worked to continue to provide a secure and loving home for them for as long as we could. But in 1987 our older son, who was then twenty-one, accidentally discovered that Gordon and I had been on a trip together. We then told him I was gay and had an ongoing relationship with Gordon. Our younger son had just left for his first year of college, and we decided not to speak with him until he returned for Christmas vacation. At the time divorce was not imminent, and we reassured them. But both boys were angry and upset, not so much at my being gay as at feeling betrayed by my secret life and by the appearance of a happy marriage. I believe our decision not to burden either them or the marriage by telling them had been correct, but I also believe that the secrecy has had the lasting effect of making them less trusting of their perceptions of their world.

The boys' knowledge undoubtedly made easier my wife's growing conviction that it was untenable for her to stay in a marriage that was making her increasingly unhappy. The next year she asked me for a divorce. I was distressed by losing someone I still cared about and had shared so much with, but I was also relieved and excited by the prospect of the future–having a more authentic life, living with Gordon, and defining new roles, socially and within my profession.

Healing Homosexuals:
A Psychologist's Journey
Through the Ex-Gay Movement
and the Pseudo-Science
of Reparative Therapy

Jeffry G. Ford, MA, LP

SUMMARY. Reparative therapy has become a generic term for any process that purports to facilitate a shift from homosexual orientation to heterosexual orientation. The author shares his own process as a survivor and former practitioner of reparative therapy. The religious mind-set and presuppositions that support reparative therapy are explored. The history of the grass roots ex-gay movement and the political ramifications associated with claims of healing are exposed. The author concludes that the pseudo-scientific claims of reparative therapy are suspect and warns of the risks and potential harm associated with these experimental therapies. *[Article copies available for a fee from The Haworth Document Delivery Service: 1-800-HAWORTH. E-mail address: <getinfo@haworthpressinc.com> Website: <http://www.HaworthPress.com> © 2001 by The Haworth Press, Inc. All rights reserved.]*

KEYWORDS. Reparative therapy, ex-gay, gay, homosexual, conversion therapy, religion, religious, Christian, Exodus International, healing, sexual orientation

Jeffry G. Ford is affiliated with Associated Resources in Psychology, P.A., Minneapolis, MN.

[Haworth co-indexing entry note]: "Healing Homosexuals: A Psychologist's Journey Through the Ex-Gay Movement and the Pseudo-Science of Reparative Therapy." Ford, Jeffry G. Co-published simultaneously in *Journal of Gay & Lesbian Psychotherapy* (The Haworth Medical Press, an imprint of The Haworth Press, Inc.) Vol. 5, No. 3/4, 2001, pp. 69-86; and: *Sexual Conversion Therapy: Ethical, Clinical and Research Perspectives* (ed: Ariel Shidlo, Michael Schroeder, and Jack Drescher) The Haworth Medical Press, an imprint of The Haworth Press, Inc., 2001, pp. 69-86. Single or multiple copies of this article are available for a fee from The Haworth Document Delivery Service [1-800-HAWORTH, 9:00 a.m. - 5:00 p.m. (EST). E-mail address: getinfo@haworthpressinc.com].

69

This article is, by its nature, subjective. I am sharing my experience and perspectives as one who was heavily involved in the ex-gay movement. I have since become a psychologist and offer my views based on my experience, the scientific literature on changing sexual orientation and an active caseload of clients affected by the experience of having attempted conversion therapies.

My story is similar to some gay men raised during the 1960s. I didn't enjoy rough and tumble play. I tended to enjoy the company of girls more than boys. I played with dolls and enjoyed dressing up in mom's clothes. In the beginning my parents and other adults found it amusing but as it continued I became aware of their concern and anxiety. By the age of 13, I was fantasizing sexually about men and boys. My mother was aware of my attractions and behavior. She caught me masturbating and playing naked with a neighbor boy. Her response let me know she was very sickened by it and considered me to be deviant. She had our pediatrician talk to me and forbade me from having any further contact with the neighbor boy.

My father was a gentle and compassionate man. He spent hours with me playing cards and board games. I always felt loved and accepted by him. He frequently verbalized how proud he was of me. I was unable to explain to him the feelings I was experiencing. When other guys at school were trying to "feel up" girls, I was noticing the developing muscles and facial hair on the boys. I frequently tried to arrange opportunities so I could be in the locker room when the athletes were showering. I felt profoundly aroused and profoundly ashamed. I knew of no other boys who were like me. I remember crying about it late at night in my bed. Everything in my environment confirmed my greatest fears. There were no examples of healthy gay males. I believe I was conditioned by my environment to feel self-hatred, inferiority and weakness.

In high school I became determined to hide my true feelings and to try to become "normal." I dated several girls and learned to brag about my heterosexual dalliances. I did "feel up" girls and tried to become aroused by looking at my brother's *Playboy* magazines. Inevitably I would spend hours looking through old issues trying to find images of men which would occasionally appear in the "History of Sex" or "Sex in the Cinema" features of the magazine. As a church-going adolescent, I found myself begging God to make this all go away. When I was 17 I became a born-again Christian and studied the Bible with fundamentalist believers.

As a fundamentalist, a personal relationship with Jesus Christ is emphasized. A very literal and legalistic interpretation of scripture is espoused. Scripture is viewed as literal truth without error and to be trusted far more than one's own subjective or intellectual senses. There are moral absolutes, some of which, if broken, without repentance, lead to eternal damnation. There are spoken and unspoken rules that govern the acceptability of certain persons as true Christians. There is an emphasis on conformity. Acceptance with good standing is dependent on obedience. Sexual activity of any kind, outside the bonds of heterosexual marriage, is seen as sinful. Homosexuality is forbidden and seen as a perversion. At the same time, fundamentalist Christians frequently emphasize the unconditional love of God. As a closeted homosexual deeply in denial, I wanted somehow to find acceptance and love.

The feelings of defectiveness and isolation made me vulnerable to accept the very conditional and demanding love offered by religious fundamentalism. This began my decade-long search for sexual healing in what has come to be know as the ex-gay or reparative therapy movement. Reparative therapy has become a generic term for almost any approach to healing homosexuality. Reparative therapy always starts with the presupposition that homosexuality is defective and sinful. Before I continue sharing my history and involvement, I want to lay a groundwork to familiarize the reader with the allure of reparative therapy.

Reparative therapy offers the fundamentalist homosexual a way to acknowledge his sexual and affectional feelings without fear of rejection. Seeking reparative therapy is seen as evidence of obedience and willingness to submit to God and Scripture. Frequently these individuals experience a great deal of love and support from others who have come out as struggling ex-gays admitting to their own sexual imperfection. The love and acceptance the homosexual fundamentalist finds within the ex-gay movement is liberating. To move from feeling isolated and alone into a community where others have shared a similar life experience is overwhelming. It is right up there with falling in love or tasting chocolate for the first time.

The ex-gay movement dates back to the mid 1970s, coinciding with the post-Stonewall gay liberation movement. Prior to this time, fundamentalist homosexuals were closeted as much or more than their mainstream counterparts.

The concept of reparative therapy was introduced by the British academic, Elizabeth Moberly, in the early 1980s. Since that time numerous Christian fundamentalist psychotherapists have adopted the term. A variety of books and periodicals have been published promoting the theory. Proponents of reparative therapy assert that homosexuality is pathological and stems from a breakdown in the relationship of the child with the same-sex parent. It is assumed that by meeting the unmet needs of these "wounded" homosexuals, their true identity and orientation as heterosexuals will emerge. I will address reparative therapy in greater detail later in the article. (It is beyond the scope of this article to address the specific claims of reparative therapists and the lack of documented evidence supporting its efficacy.)

Men and women in heterosexual marriages who are homosexual are especially prone to the allure of reparative therapy. I have found that, frequently, the love and communication in mixed gay/straight marriages are healthy and strong. It is the sexual passion and fulfillment that is missing. The promise of healing by submitting to counseling can seem tempting because it allows for what is already good in the marriage to continue. Given that society at large still does not affirm and support the integration and celebration of one's homosexual identity, the path of least resistance often appears to be conformity.

Persons seeking reparative therapy are almost always very religious with an ideology that precludes accepting or integrating their homosexuality. When a gay man or lesbian first encounter the promises of a changed life and freedom from self-hatred and societal oppression, there is a profound sense of relief and hopefulness. When interacting with them on an individual basis, ex-gay ministries and reparative therapy counselors are generally very warm and accepting. They do not focus on the sinfulness and depravity of the homosexual condition. Instead, they tend to normalize homosexual feelings as something common to men and women who have had tough childhoods and lack of connection and support from their same sex parent. This acceptance is something akin to the acceptance a gay individual feels upon entering a gay bar or other situation where one is surrounded by a majority of gay men and lesbians. The difference however is that the love and acceptance offered by ex-gays and fundamentalists come at an extraordinary cost.

The ex-gay movement has many of the trappings that are common to strict religious sects or cults. The followers are sincere and devout; they believe what they are saying with their heart, mind and soul. There is an ex-gay theology that is in common from group to group across the country and internationally. Most believe the Bible is the ultimate authority on every issue and is the inerrant word of God. They believe homosexuality is evidence of man's sinful nature and that continuing in genital homosexual relationships will exclude one from heaven. They believe that faith in Jesus Christ is the only hope for salvation and ultimate healing from homosexuality. They believe they have "the truth" and are thus bound to share it with the world with hopes of saving some from the hell fires of perdition. Many discourage followers from associating with unbelievers thus creating separateness and single-mindedness. Followers are discouraged from reading anything written from a pro-gay perspective. To question or doubt is seen as evidence of weak faith and a potential source of opening for the enemy to penetrate.

Central to their belief system is the concept of a literal hell and Satan. This personified spirit of evil is omnipresent and capable of inhabiting the body and influencing thoughts and feelings. Temptations are seen as the work of the devil. Giving in to homosexual fantasies or behavior is seen as surrendering to Satan. There is forgiveness and grace for the repentant sinner but it is frequently mixed with shaming and chastisement. There is a profound sense of love and belonging for those who follow the rules but woe to those who stray.

Since genuine acceptance is something gay, lesbian, bisexual and transgender (GLBT) persons frequently lack but desperately crave, the ex-gay movement is especially dangerous to youth and vulnerable adults. It is my impression that, similar to other cults, the membership appears to be heavily weighted with those we might refer to as disenfranchised or at risk. Since acceptance is conditional there is strong motivation for members to report what is expected and to deny subjective experience. Feelings are always seen as suspect. To trust one's own intuition is seen as carnal and dangerous. Paradoxically, relying on intellect is also risky and frequently seen as a lack of faith. The emphasis is placed on accepting the truth as it is taught within the group. Questions are answered by elders or other leaders.

The excitement of finding other like-minded people offering hope and acceptance is intoxicating. It can surely be described as "coming home." The single-minded purpose and upbeat meetings reinforce the feelings of elation. At this point in the process, the new convert feels safe and by power of suggestion alone, may genuinely believe their sexual orientation has been changed.

The problems occur later when the newness and excitement begin to fade and the honeymoon draws to an end. The realization that those old familiar feelings are once again knocking is disarming. The convert feels she or he has done something wrong. At this point, if the ex-gay is open with the others about these feelings, they are often met with words of cautious reassurance. They might be told that the temptations are evidence that the enemy is not pleased. The concept of spiritual warfare may be explained as a huge battle taking place for the soul of the believer. "Just as Jesus was tempted in the wilderness so also the ex-gay must expect a time of testing and temptation."

There is a strong sense of martyrdom among many of those in the ex-gay reparative therapy movement. By seeing the return of homoerotic desires as an attack, the convert can disown them as something outside of themselves. This reinforces the process of repression and sublimation. A psychological splitting occurs between the good and righteous self and evil and depraved enemy. An essential component of ex-gay theology is the belief that one's heart and soul, which they refer to as "the flesh," are fallen and easily influenced by evil. The ex-gay convert is taught that the homoerotic feelings are a lie and deception. They are explained away by the reparative therapy theory as eroticized desires for legitimate love and attachment they did not receive from their mother or father.

When one has been involved with an ex-gay group for an extended period of time, there is less group tolerance for perceived failures. If an ex-gay convert repeatedly confesses to impure thoughts and sinful behaviors, like masturbation, their sincerity and faithfulness are questioned. It is perceived that there is something seriously wrong in the person's relationship with God. The blame lies not with the failure of the reparative therapist or the ex-gay group, but with the individual.

Frequently the ex-gay struggler will accept full responsibility and try harder to "get it right." The risk for depression and self-destructive thoughts and behaviors is particularly great during this phase. The person internalizes the shame and believes they are defective. They may think, if God is healing the others, "What's wrong with me?" The fear of losing the love, respect and acceptance of the group and therapist seem overwhelming. The fear of abandonment intensifies. This commonly leads to an inner awareness that it is no longer safe to tell the truth. To gain the conditional love and acceptance the ex-gay struggler must "go underground" with the existence of their ongoing homosexual attractions. Now, the person is not only a failure, they are lying about it. A cognitive dissonance occurs whereby they have strongly held beliefs but their behavior is incongruent. Holding strongly to certain moral imperatives but failing to adhere to them can create psychological confusion and depression.

To the outsider, all of this may seem hard to comprehend. There can be a tendency among self-accepting gays and lesbians to question how or why anyone could get caught up in this kind of thinking. The ex-gay struggler often feels judged and misunderstood by the GLBT community. They are frequently met with pat answers and disdain from those who have little understanding about the intensity of the internal conflict the person is experiencing. This leaves the ex-gay feeling completely isolated and trapped. They perceive the church, the ex-gay, and the GLBT communities to be unsafe. It is the intensity of these feelings and a profound sense of isolation that can cause a person to consider suicide a viable option.

The beliefs of the fundamentalist ex-gay are complex and deeply held. I will stop short of saying they have been brainwashed but the similarities among cult survivors and former ex-gays is striking. For the ex-gay to admit they are not healed and that their need and desire for homosexual contact is as strong as it ever was, is extremely humbling. They risk and often face rejection from friends and family they have loved deeply. They believe themselves to be quitters and, sadly, they believe they have been abandoned by God and face eternity in hell.

The ex-gay struggler who ventures in to the GLBT community should be embraced like a wounded soldier returning from a prisoner of war camp. They will need time to adjust and find their place. This is not a time to debate with them about their long held beliefs and ongoing fears. The ex-gay struggler should be embraced with true unconditional love. The rainbow flag of diversity must include these people as well. The GLBT community must not demand that they exchange one set of rigid rules and expectations for another. They must be allowed and even encouraged to doubt and to question whatever seems wrong, unfair or unjust. In the zeal to expose the lies and abuses perpetrated by many on the political and religious right one must be clear that it is the homophobic ideology being opposed, not the people. Ex-gay strugglers must know they are not hated. GLBT persons should be the first to understand how trapped and wounded these individuals are. The challenging process of coming out and celebrating one's sexual diversity, and refusing to accept the shame and condemnation of the majority, is common to all GLBT persons.

My own personal path toward reparative therapy continued from my high school religious conversion as I pursued conservative Christian fellowship in college. During my time at the University of Northern Colorado, I became very active in Campus Crusade for Christ and other bible studies. I met and socialized primarily with other Christians. Since I had successfully had girlfriends in high school, I convinced myself that the homosexual feelings were diminishing. I had no problems socializing with women and I enjoyed them as friends. I found I could talk and share feelings much more freely with women. At some level I started to think that marriage would be a good thing for me. I thought God would continue to take away the homosexual feelings if I had a wife who would provide a legitimate outlet for my sexual desires.

I had grown quite close to a woman in one of the Bible studies. She and I shared a mutual love and respect. In many ways we appeared an unlikely couple. I was from an upper-middle class family, raised by "proper" Episcopalian parents in metropolitan Phoenix. She was the oldest of 10 children from a family of modest means, raised on a farm in rural Iowa. She and I never really dated, but we spent almost all of our free time together. During my sophomore year and her senior year we began to talk about the future. She had hopes of going on full-time staff with Campus Crusade or entering the mission field in some capacity. I think it was the idea of losing my best friend, more than an erotic and romantic type of love, that led me to propose marriage.

Our mutual friends thought it was quite a hoot when we announced our engagement. Most of them were aware we had never even shared a passionate kiss. It is hard to know for sure what I was thinking or feeling so many years ago. I do recall how awkward and weird it felt when we started to introduce sexual intimacy into our relationship. I secretly prayed for God's will and for his healing. Up until this point I had never told anyone about my sexual orientation. I wrestled internally with the decision not to tell my future wife about it. I was desperately afraid of her rejection. I was equally convinced that since I had never embraced a gay identity and, aside from some high school experimentation, had never acted on my homosexual urges, that I wasn't really gay. This is a decision I deeply regret. Although the outcome may have been the same, given the depth of my denial, my deception robbed Cathy of her right to freely choose. With absence of malice, I trapped her into a situation that eventually brought her a tremendous amount of pain. As with most things in life, it's not all black or white. We shared many good times together, and as a result of our union we were blessed with the opportunity to share in the lives of two very precious children.

It was just over two years into our marriage before I told my wife about my secret struggle. We had moved to Phoenix and I had dropped out of college to run my brother's insurance agency. It was a busy first year of marriage. We bought a small condominium, started new jobs, and got involved in a local Evangelical church. On the surface everything appeared to be going well. Inside, it was another story.

The all too familiar feelings and desires had returned. I think I was pretty discouraged and angry with God. I felt I had been obedient by trusting God's direction and getting married. I saw no reason why God would have me continue to battle this demon. I felt like a failure especially because I had yielded to temptation and bought a *Playgirl* magazine. It was absolutely erotic and exciting to look at the pictures. These were feelings I was not having with my wife, and I remember thinking about past encounters I had experienced with high school friends. I could not understand why God would not just "fix" whatever was broken. I continued through prayer to beg God to make me normal.

A friend of ours came to visit us shortly after our first anniversary. He had been the best man in our wedding. He was a friend from my childhood who had frequently encouraged me in my Christian faith. He had been my counselor at an Inter-Varsity Christian Fellowship summer camp. He and I went camping in the White Mountains of northern Arizona. He was perceptive and could tell that all was not well with me. I'm not sure to this day why but after 21 years of silence, he became the first person with whom I shared my secret. He thought the pressures of living around my family and starting such a challenging career were putting too much stress on me. He minimized the significance of what he viewed as temptations and encouraged me not to start thinking I was gay. He also suggested I might be happier back in a college setting but this time on a Christian campus in the Midwest. He said there would be trained counselors I could talk to in confidence.

Without telling Cathy about my homosexual feelings, I suggested that living in Phoenix was not a good thing for me. She was not liking it much either and welcomed the idea of going back to the Midwest, much closer to her family and friends. Upon gaining acceptance at Bethel, we announced to my family that we were moving to Minnesota. This announcement was met first with shock and later with disapproval. We crammed everything we owned into the back of a U-Haul trailer and drove in tandem from Phoenix to St. Paul.

We got settled into a small one-bedroom apartment. I began taking classes and Cathy took a job with a mortgage company in downtown St. Paul. Several months after enrolling, I finally got the courage to sign up for an appointment with a handsome counselor from the psychology department. My journal entries from this time in my life are telling.

From My Journal, March 28, 1978

I am going to meet with the counselor tomorrow. I don't really know what to think. I feel that I need help but I also feel that I'm trying to do away with a part of myself. I know I should look at it as sinful and ugly, like a wart that needs to be burned off. Is it possible that those emotions are what allow me to be a sensitive caring male? Is it possible that God has allowed this in my life to build certain characteristics? Is it really ugly and sinful that I want to hold and be held by a man and that I want to have a relationship with a man that includes sex? It sure sounds ugly on paper. I don't like admitting these things. I really don't. What is it that causes me to think and feel this way? Is it Satanic? Am I possessed? Where does Cathy fit in? How can I love her as much as I do and do this to her? I am so torn by my emotions. I wish both parts of me could live within my one body. I love Cathy more than anyone else on earth. I don't want to hurt her. Oh Lord, I don't want her hurt! What would she do? What would she think if she found out about me?

This entry shows only the tip of the internal torment and confusion I was experiencing. I was married to a woman I cared for deeply. I wanted to please God. I wanted to be true to myself. I was agonizing over it. My experience is not unique. Ex-gay strugglers sincerely desire and attempt to live by their convictions. Central to the process is the presumption that they are defective, broken, sinful and unacceptable. This internalized homophobia is supported and reinforced by society, religion, family and friends.

I met with the psychologist. He was kind and supportive. He assured me there were others at Bethel facing similar temptations. It was comforting to know others were out there but due to confidentiality concerns he could not put us in touch. Dr. A. took a cognitive behavioral approach. After gathering family and sexual history, he suggested I would be a good candidate for a procedure known as aversive conditioning.

The process of aversive conditioning or electric shock therapy involves pairing negative stimuli "shock" with the unwanted psychosexual response. In my case, I was frequently hooked up to an additional device known as a penile plythysmograph used to measure blood engorgement to the penis. When the meter shows arousal, the shock is immediately administered. In theory, for this to be effective there must be a strong arousal. I was invited to look through stacks of homosexual pornography to identify images that would be particularly effective for that purpose. The sessions lasted about 45 to 50 minutes during which dozens of shocks were administered. The two electrodes strapped to the underside of my forearm left burn marks the size of quarters.

The psychologist also used a therapy known as covert sensitization. During these sessions I was encouraged to imagine a very stimulating same-sex encounter. As I experienced strong arousal I was guided into a scenario that was either repulsive or frightening. On one occasion the object of my attraction vomited all over me. On another occasion I was arrested by an undercover police officer. The combined therapies spanned about 40 sessions over a three or four month period of time.

During the period of time when I was actually going through the weekly therapies, I recall feeling hopeful and reported that I was having far fewer homosexual fantasies. As treatment progressed and the time between appointments was being stretched out, the fantasies started to increase. Within a month or so of termination, the fantasies were back to pre-treatment levels if not greater.

The process, in my opinion, was barbaric and abusive. I felt ashamed and embarrassed waiting in the outer office with patients of other therapists. I would try to hide my arm or wear long sleeve shirts so others wouldn't see the burn marks as I left. The emotional roller coaster was fatiguing. I sank into depression when I realized the painful and expensive therapy had failed.

From My Journal, July 2, 1979

> I am not finding the victory that I portray on the outside. I feel that I am living a lie. I have many things to work through in my life. I am in no way "under control." Lord, which way do I turn? How hard do I have to try before your grace will intervene? Is the ex-gay life no different than a celibate homosexual lifestyle? God, where is the freedom? Are we following the wrong path? Do you honestly want people to remain in bondage to homosexual temptation? Lord, what are we going to do about this situation? You know how much I love Cathy. You also know how I look at men and what I long for. God, it's out of my hands, it's up to you. My own wisdom and insight is not sufficient to handle this situation. How can I tell others that Jesus offers help for the homosexual when I am not healed? I don't want you to look bad so I put on a front. How long can this go on? I know that the testing of my faith produces endurance but this is getting to be ridiculous!! Why do homosexuals have to go through so much hell? Is it a handicap or some sort of cross to bare? Dearest Triune God, I ask you to reveal the truth to me in a very real and very dynamic way. If you will honor this request, I will share the truth with as many as will listen, by any means that you will provide. I am a Christian. I accept Jesus as Lord and Savior of my life. I lay claim to the promises that are mine. Lord you must answer my prayer. Convict my heart and show me your truth. Just for the record, I want to be free from all homo-

sexual temptation and sin. I want to be healed, if this is what healing is, but I refuse to lie. I must know genuine healing and God's unblemished truth or I can't go on. Speak to me soon Lord God, speak to me now. These things I pray in the name of Jesus Christ, the Son of God, who died to set me free. Amen!

I hope as you read the words from my journal you can sense the intensity and sincerity of my struggle. I know from my years within the ex-gay movement that the desire to love and serve God is genuine. Ex-gay followers and leaders are, in most instances, very good people trying to do what they believe is God's will. When I wrote "or I can't go on" in the journal entry above, I was referring to suicide. The idea of accepting myself as a gay man was impossible for me to comprehend. The mindset of the ex-gay struggler cannot accept or integrate the possibility of being gay and Christian at the same time. The thought of living my life as a gay man and going to hell seemed much worse than taking my own life while I was still in grace.

When aversive conditioning didn't work, I went in search of what else might be out there. I read every new Christian book on the subject. I joined the counseling staff at OUTPOST, a Minneapolis based ex-gay ministry, and as a result was able to communicate with people across the country and overseas. The original intent of the annual Exodus conference was to provide an opportunity for other like-minded people to share information and fellowship. Keynote speakers were brought in to share the latest ideas on homosexual healing and recovery.

Within the ex-gay movement, there was division and controversy over the role of "demons" and the sin of homosexuality. Some believed that by exorcism or deliverance, the demon of homosexuality could be cast out affording the believer an instantaneous cure. When temptations returned or persisted the victim of the exorcist was often blamed. The concept of "secret sin" was introduced. It was assumed unsuccessful exorcisms were the result of sin that had not been confessed. After episodes of deliverance or exorcism, which were frequently long and dramatic, there was tremendous psychological pressure to report healing. I don't think the reports of healing were deliberate attempts to deceive. The emotional intensity of the experience, the expectation for change, and the peer pressure all worked together to reinforce the denial. The emphasis on this form of healing has lessened considerably over the years. The evidence of radically changed lives was never there to support it.

My deliverance experience was not particularly remarkable. I sought out a charismatic Lutheran minister in the Twin Cities and requested help. There was no screaming or frothing at the mouth. The minister laid his hands on me at the altar of the church and asked me to "renounce Satan in all his works and all his ways." He spoke in tongues for awhile and declared me healed. He exhorted me to claim my healing by faith. He warned, if I entertained homosexual thoughts again, I would be opening the door for seven more demons to enter where the one had left. Apart from being scared out of my wits, my experience with exorcism was not life changing.

As a movement, the emphasis moved away from immediate healing and shifted to discipleship model. Healing is seen as a process and an event. This conceptual change allows ex-gay devotees to honestly say they are healed even though homosexual attractions persist. A common battle cry or slogan of the ex-gay crowd is "by His stripes we are healed." The healing is seen as something already accomplished by Jesus. The role of the disciple is to "name it and claim it." A national leader and cofounder of Homosexuals Anonymous, Colin Cook, espoused a complex theology. Based in his exegesis from the New Testament book of Romans, Cook taught that everyone is heterosexual in Christ. This concept aids in the believer's struggle with duplicity. The ex-gay sees heterosexuality as something they can claim as true while viewing homosexuality as a deception. The newest ex-gay covert, snatched from Satan's grasp out of a homosexual love affair, can honestly say, "I am heterosexual" or "I am straight" while reframing homosexual attractions as illusory and untrue.

Cook developed an extensive training seminar that was required before a Homosexuals Anonymous group could be established. The OUTPOST Board approved a motion allowing the ministry to provide space and resources for a local HA chapter to begin. I was chosen to go to Reading, PA for the week-long training. While in Reading I stayed with Colin and Sharon Cook and their two children. Cook became for me a role model and hero. He seemed to have a handle on the ex-gay theology and had achieved a level of healing I had not seen anywhere else. Cook told me he was 100% heterosexual and had the answers to help others achieve the same. I took copious notes at the seminar and bought his 10-tape series on overcoming homosexuality.

Homosexuals Anonymous groups are self-led. There is no paid staff. The only requirement for membership is a desire to be free from homosexuality. It is a 14-step group that closely resembles the format of Alcoholics Anonymous. Cook reworded many of the steps to make them specifically Christian and added a couple of new steps as well. I was so impressed with Colin Cook I invited him to keynote for the annual OUTPOST two-day workshop. Ministry leaders from around the country came to hear Cook for the first time. His insistence that God had completely healed him was unique in the ex-gay movement at that time.

Cook's bold proclamations were soon to be exposed as lies. Members of a pro-gay Adventist group known as Kinship got word that some of his clients reported having received nude massages from Cook during the course of therapy. Kinship members interviewed dozens of his former clients. Seventh-Day Adventist sociologist Ronald Lawson uncovered evidence from 14 young men who complained of sexual pressures from Cook during counseling sessions.

On November 19, 1987 the board of Cook's Quest Learning Center/Homosexuals Anonymous voted to accept his resignation and to close Quest. It decided to continue HA in a new location and with services limited primarily to mail and phone contact rather than face-to-face counseling.

Cook used his position of power to manipulate vulnerable men and objectify them for his own self-gratification. He appeared on the Phil Donahue Show earlier in 1987 proclaiming the ex-gay message. Even after the producers were informed of Cook's resignation and misdeeds, they rebroadcast the show on December 19, 1987. I had been privy to numerous rumors and anecdotal stories about Colin years prior to the public announcement. Cook's story is not unique. Ex-gay leaders and followers frequently engage in homosexual contact. It was this awareness that led my wife and I to seriously question the honesty of the message we were proclaiming.

Inner healing is a form of prayer therapy used by many ex-gay practitioners. It involves a prayerful guided imagery experience during which the Holy Spirit is invited to reveal unresolved hurt and woundedness in the life of the ex-gay subject. Unlike deliverance or exorcism, the inner healing experience tends to be soothing. In my persistent pursuit of healing, I became enamored with the teachings of Leanne Payne. She is the author of several books on inner healing. She was brought in by Exodus to keynote at one of their annual conferences. She is just one among many figureheads whose ideas were popularized for a period of time only to be replaced or accessorized with the next "concept de jour." My wife and I attended her workshops and conferences and devoured her books. I contacted her in confidence and requested a private consultation. Since I was a respected leader in the ex-gay movement, she consented. I was invited to her home in Milwaukee. Once again, I got my hopes up, believing God was going to answer my heartfelt prayer for healing.

From My Journal, December 11, 1983

> Met with Leanne Payne. Shared my dream about the tiger chasing me into my parents backyard and other history. She saw both characters in my dream as being me. She saw me as being separated from my own masculinity and putting my masculine self in great danger. She prayed and anointed me with oil. She saw "darts" in my mind, lies that had entered in. She had me deal with bitterness and unforgiveness toward my mother. I saw fear in my mind, fear of someone hurting me or beating me up. Jesus helped me pull out that weed and he burned it. . . . We prayed through my envy and insecurity with my body. Her advice for me is to live from the center, to no longer walk along side of myself. My homosexual desires are just a desire to love myself. I am projecting my masculinity onto another person, unable to accept it in myself. She prayed that I

would write and become an author. She anointed my hands with oil as she prayed. She says the healing is complete. My mother has been healed and freed and so has Rick B. She says in relation to K. that I may discover a whole new way to love him as a man. This lasted 2 hours. No intense emotion but some tears did come. By faith I claim the healing and I will walk by faith in the completed work of Jesus Christ.

Once again, my hopes were raised but to no avail. I kept on trying to understand and accept the inner healing that was to have taken place. A year or two later Payne's next book *Crisis In Masculinity* came out. I was shocked and saddened to see she had used me as one of her examples without ever having asked my permission. The concept of boundaries and professionalism is frequently lacking within the para-church ex-gay ministries. Most of the "counselors" have no professional training.

My own ignorance about boundaries emerged when I formed an intimate friendship with a member of the local HA group. We were instantly drawn to one another. I was sexually attracted to him. It wasn't long before we had our first "fall." Here was another occasion that brought me to a place of desperation. He and I felt tremendous guilt about our sexual experiences together. It was so confusing. I felt emotion and attraction toward him I had never experienced with my wife. The intensity of the sexual experience was remarkable. The intensity of the guilt was almost unbearable.

We felt compelled to confess our sins to my wife. She was understandably quite upset. She didn't want to know the details. She said she felt betrayed and disrespected. She also felt it was not her place to tell me what to do about it. She was hurt and frustrated by the lack of genuine "healing" taking place in my life. She was also aware my situation was not unique. As leaders in the ex-gay movement, we were privy to inside information about numerous "falls" and indiscretions taking place across the country. It was not uncommon for members of the Board of Directors for Exodus to be disciplined or removed as a result of sexual acting out.

After a great deal of prayer and conversation, Cathy and I decided to continue to try to make things work. We had just adopted a child. We were financially dependent on the ministry for survival. We put all of our chips on one last glimmer of hope. Elizabeth Moberly's reparative therapy model was presented as science. Moberly's writings sounded intelligent and articulate. I used my influence as an ex-gay leader and along with Robbie Kenney, the founder of Outpost, and Doug Houck, the founder of Metanoia Ministries in Seattle, WA, we contacted Dr. Moberly in Great Britain. We offered to bring her to the States to present conferences on her theory. Cathy and I became friends with her and invited her into our home. She was convinced that as my legitimate same-sex love needs were met, my homosexual attractions would abate. Based on this theoretical assumption, my wife encouraged me to continue in my relationship with the HA member, albeit without further sexual involvement. The goal of course was healing.

I found myself falling in love with a beautiful man. I went back into therapy with the same Christian psychologist who had attempted the aversive conditioning. I told him everything and had him read Moberly's book *Homosexuality: A New Christian Ethic*. For many months Kent, my HA friend (and now partner of 12+ years) and I tried to affirm each other's masculinity. We attempted to keep the relationship above reproach. My therapist was also very supportive and nurturing. We were doing our best to see if reparative therapy would work.

Instead of the erotic desires diminishing, they seemed to become more intense. Instead of feeling better about myself as a heterosexual, I was beginning to like and accept myself as a gay man. In addition to reading Moberly's book, I was also reading *The Road Less Traveled* by M. Scott Peck. I was impressed by Peck's premise that "Life is difficult." I was especially challenged by his call to live life with honesty and integrity. I was confused for a period of time. I was trying to figure out, as Peck encouraged, what it meant for me to accept responsibility and face the truth.

I looked back on the years of tormented struggle doing what I thought was God's will. I pondered the realities I was aware of within the greater ex-gay movement. I continued to pray and seek God's will. I became convinced I needed to face the pain of rejection, financial loss, and uncertainty about my marriage and the future. I discontinued my therapy for a while and took a leave of absence from the ministry. Kent and I privately affirmed our love and commitment to one another and to God in prayer. Six months after going before the Board of Directors and explaining the truth about my love and relationship with Kent, I offered my resignation.

My wife stayed on with the ministry for another year but she knew also she would need to find another means of employment. It took a few more years of therapy with gay affirming therapists for all of us to reconcile with ourselves and each other. Cathy and I separated and Kent and I moved in together. We agreed to share joint physical and legal custody of the children. For the past 12 years we have lived only blocks away from my ex-wife. We have shared all major holidays and birthday celebrations together as a family. When we divorced, we did not stop loving one another. We chose to redefine our relationship to reflect what it was from the beginning, a deeply committed friendship.

I think the single greatest challenge facing the conflicted ex-gay struggler is the decision to emancipate. Emancipation is a necessary stage of emotional development for all adolescents and young adults. During emancipation, adolescents and young adults challenge the boundaries and beliefs set forth parents, teachers, ministers and others who have held a place of authority in their lives. During this time adolescents and young adults will explore: their sexual feelings and beliefs, their political leanings, their religious convictions and so much more. This is a necessary phase in healthy development of self-esteem and autonomy. Adolescents who are allowed and encouraged to think for themselves and explore doubts or questions gradually foreclose on a sense of self identity. This is an evolutionary process that changes and develops over time. Psychologically healthy people are always evolving, taking in new information and integrating it as necessary.

Based on my personal experience as an ex-gay leader and my clinical experience treating survivors of ex-gay groups, it appears to me that many ex-gay persons may experience challenges with issues of emancipation and autonomy. They tend to look to people in authority to help define them. They are often taught not to trust their own instincts. They become convinced that, due to their sinful brokenness, they cannot trust or believe in themselves. Since they lack the ability to think and make decisions on their own, they are quite prone to become followers of charismatic leaders or movements. They prefer a world where black and white, right and wrong are clearly defined for them. They cannot tolerate the anxiety associated with unknowns. Since they may have little internalized sense of safety and self-confidence, they tend to rely on beliefs and dogma which are clear and distinct.

When the ex-gay struggler admits to his or her defective sinfulness, fundamentalist Christians are quick to confirm this and offer strict guidelines and conditional acceptance. As with many religious cults and fundamentalist sects, ex-gays develop a victim mentality. A sense of martyrdom is assumed. The internal suffering is perceived to be a "cross to bear." Rather than embracing and accepting themselves, ex-gays look forward to the next life when they will be rewarded for their faithfulness.

There is a strong sense of community and support among ex-gays. However, there is an ever present guardedness that prevails lest one become emotionally dependent or sexually attracted to a fellow struggler. It is this very dilemma that continues to challenge the ex-gay movement. When gay Christians were closeted and isolated, there was little opportunity for "slips and falls." By bringing them together, the ex-gay movement has had to deal with the "temptation" that comes when one is in the presence of the object of lust or desire.

Ex-gay groups vary in their approach to handling concerns about sexual or emotional transgression among members. Most attempt to regulate or control it by the imposition of rules and guidelines. For instance, it is seen as improper for two ex-gays to be alone with one another. They are encouraged to meet and fellowship in groups of three or more. Friendships that are becoming too intense are broken up or at least contact is significantly curtailed.

There are some things that can be potentially very comforting and healthy about the ex-gay ministries. Due to being a minority within a minority, ex-gay

Christians often form very meaningful connections with one another. Since sexual relationships are strictly forbidden, these men and women are forced to relate to one another first on an emotional and psychological level. The sexual tension is constant, but by sheer strength of will or fear they frequently refrain from consummating the relationship. These friendships develop over time based on a sense of genuine care and respect. This is why the pain of separation and sexual repression becomes so intense.

When ex-gay friendships are allowed to continue, they often become the needed motivator that jump starts the dormant or repressed drive for emancipation. The subjective experience of falling in love is extremely intense. Many ex-gays and gays alike report it was experiencing the strong emotional bond with a same-sex person that precipitated the decision to "come out." A thought something like "How can something that seems this right be so wrong?" encourages the process of self appraisal. This can lead to greater emancipation and eventual foreclosure on a homosexual identity. Since the term *reparative therapy* is a generic descriptor for a variety of ex-gay modalities, the relative dangers and side-effects vary from practitioner to practitioner. Former ex-gays report having experiences that range from relatively benign to intensely destructive.

The political aspect of the ex-gay movement cannot be ignored nor should it be minimized. There is a very strong, well-organized and well-financed mechanism in place to systematically repeal gay rights ordinances, to get the pseudo science of reparative therapy into the schools and to influence public opinion toward homophobic polarization. By creating ex-gay "superstars" to parade before the media and political decision makers, they hope to stir up just enough doubt and concern to sway the "malleable middle" toward the "repressive right."

I reflect on my years in the ex-gay movement with varied emotions. At the time, I believed I was doing the right thing. I felt we were pioneers. In time the ex-gay movement will form a unique piece of the greater mosaic in GLBT history. I feel grief and responsibility for the misguided direction I offered many sincere and wonderful people. I continue to trust in the sovereignty of God and believe all things work together for good. I am so fortunate to have a loving partner and beautiful kids. Our neighbors and schools have been kind and supportive. The peace and wholeness I am experiencing make the challenges and difficulties of the *road less traveled* all worthwhile.

I urge psychologists and all psychotherapists to expose the pseudo-science of reparative therapy. I encourage all licensed professionals to pressure their respective Boards to address the ethical concerns and psychological dangers associated with this experimental therapy. I invite victims of reparative therapy to come forward and pursue legal and psychological remedies. I am aware of numerous attorneys who are actively encouraging those wounded by reparative therapy to hold their professional perpetrators liable.

What started as a grass roots movement led by religious GLBT persons has been taken over by extremists from the religious and political right. Their clear and stated goals involve changing public opinion and so called special protection under the law. They use unsupported claims from the pseudo-science of reparative therapy to further their cause.

Although my partner and I survived our years in the ex-gay movement, I would not wish them on anyone. I will sound the alarm concerning the social implications of what has become a multimillion dollar organized campaign to spread misinformation for political gain. I will continue to do anything in my power to expose their fraudulent claims.

Cures versus Choices:
Agendas in Sexual Reorientation Therapy

A. Lee Beckstead, PhD

SUMMARY. Longstanding debates have occurred in the mental health fields on the issues surrounding sexual reorientation therapy. Both sides agree that a subset of individuals with same-sex attractions seeks help or a "cure" for their homosexual attractions. However, each position tends to respond with a limited, exclusionary choice to be an "out" gay or an "ex"-gay. These dichotomized options may not serve all clients with same-sex attractions who are seeking help in dealing with religious conflicts. The perspectives of 20 individuals (2 women, 18 men) who reported benefiting from reparative/conversion therapy are described. In contrast to previous imprecise claims of change, a more complex conceptual framework is presented regarding the definitions of a successful outcome from such treatments. Research and political implications are discussed as well as the need for more effective clinical strategies that integrate conservative social identities with same-sex attractions. *[Article copies available for a fee from The Haworth Document Delivery Service: 1-800-HAWORTH. E-mail address: <getinfo@haworthpressinc.com> Website: <http://www.HaworthPress.com> © 2001 by The Haworth Press, Inc. All rights reserved.]*

A. Lee Beckstead is affiliated with the University of Utah, Department of Educational Psychology.

Address correspondence to: A. Lee Beckstead, 1705 East Campus Center Drive, Room 327, Salt Lake City, UT 84112-9255 (E-mail: leebeckst@yahoo.com).

The author gives acknowledgment to Lynda Brzezinski, Sue Morrow, James Cantor, and Ariel Shidlo for their advice and editing.

The results presented in this paper are from the author's unpublished Master's thesis and were previously presented as a poster at the annual meeting of the American Psychological Association, Boston, MA, August 23, 1999.

[Haworth co-indexing entry note]: "Cures versus Choices: Agendas in Sexual Reorientation Therapy." Beckstead, A. Lee. Co-published simultaneously in *Journal of Gay & Lesbian Psychotherapy* (The Haworth Medical Press, an imprint of The Haworth Press, Inc.) Vol. 5, No. 3/4, 2001, pp. 87-115; and: *Sexual Conversion Therapy: Ethical, Clinical and Research Perspectives* (ed: Ariel Shidlo, Michael Schroeder, and Jack Drescher) The Haworth Medical Press, an imprint of The Haworth Press, Inc., 2001, pp. 87-115. Single or multiple copies of this article are available for a fee from The Haworth Document Delivery Service [1-800-HAWORTH, 9:00 a.m. - 5:00 p.m. (EST). E-mail address: getinfo@haworthpressinc.com].

KEYWORDS. Sexual reorientation therapy, reparative therapy, conversion therapy, homosexuality, gay, lesbian, bisexuality, religion

Sexual reorientation therapies, commonly referred to as conversion or reparative therapies, have been developed for individuals who sense themselves to be "homosexual" and find this identity incongruent. Historically, mental-health professions have offered sexual reorientation treatments that have ranged from biological, behavioral, cognitive, and psychodynamic to religious as a means for homosexuals to develop into heterosexuals (cf. Drescher, 1998a; Haldeman, 1991, 1994; LeVay, 1996; Murphy, 1992, 1997).

Current approaches tend to utilize religious and psychodynamic principles that define homosexuality as a "condition" that results when a child does not receive sufficient love through the attachment to the same-sex parent, thereby creating an estrangement toward same-sex others. Moberly (1983), for example, theorized that a gay man is like a boy who yearns for his father's love, which Moberly affirmed as a normal and valid need. However, her theoretical perspective is that this need becomes pathologically sexualized in its search for what she calls "same-sex completion." She defined adult homosexuality as "fundamentally a confusion of the emotional needs of the non-adult with the physiological desires of the adult" (p. 21). According to Nicolosi (1993), the core issue for male homosexuals is their sense of feeling different and inferior from same-sex parents and peers: "It is this internal sense of incompleteness in one's own maleness [that] is the essential foundation for homoerotic attraction" (p. 211). Female homosexuality is rarely discussed within sexual reorientation theories, although Elaine Siegel's (1988) work is a notable exception. Current sexual reorientation treatments for both sexes tend to offer "gender lessons" and support groups whereby clients can see others of the same sex as friends rather than sexual partners. With these cognitive shifts, clients theoretically can "catch up, to conquer what the heterosexual . . . achieved years before" (Nicolosi, 1993, p. 213). For the sake of salvation, sexual reorientation programs tend to rely on the power of God and prayer to help the repentant homosexual strengthen willpower, reduce desire, and limit behavior (Ritter and O'Neill, 1989). Heterosexual marriage and children are promised, which sexual reorientation therapists consider a healthy adaptation to a heterosexual world (Nicolosi, 1991). For purposes of this article, the term, "sexual reorientation therapy" is used as an umbrella category for the entire enterprise of attempting a change in sexual orientation via therapy; the terms "conversion" and "reparative" therapy are used synonymously for those treatments that are religious in nature and utilize a gender-identity etiology.

Two dichotomized clinical and political agendas have intersected around the issue of sexual reorientation. The first agenda tries to create a method of eliminating sexual attractions to same-sex individuals and to foster a hetero-sexual conversion ("gay is bad") while the second aims to promote the expression to self and others of a homosexual identity and to validate same-sex sexual and emotional relationships ("gay is good"). Corresponding with these two perspectives, institutional debates in the mental health fields have emerged that question whether to ban or further develop these treatments. The current debates parallel the historical discussions that took place during the declassification of homosexuality as a mental illness (cf. Bayer, 1981). The aim of this article is to present the two polarized perspectives of the discussions on sexual reorientation, the oversimplification felt to characterize both views, and the potential harm to clients of forcing an all-or-nothing choice to be an "out" gay or an "ex"-gay.

THE ETHICS OF SEXUAL REORIENTATION THERAPY: SELF-DETERMINATION AND EFFICACY

Among others, two issues have emerged surrounding the ethics of sexual reorientation therapy: (a) providing clients with the opportunity to self-determine and (b) evaluating the efficacy of such interventions. On the one hand, proponents of reparative therapy believe that "non-gay" homosexual clients (Nicolosi, 1991) have the right to choose the kind of therapy they receive and the freedom to choose how to live out their sexual orientation. Supporters of this argument cite the American Psychological Association's (APA) General Principle D of the Ethics Code (APA, 1992), which calls for "Respect for People's Rights and Dignity" and affirms that psychologists be aware of and respect cultural and individual differences. Both religion and sexual orientation are among these differences. Furthermore, Standard 1.09 expects that "psychologists respect the rights of others to hold values, attitudes, and opinions that differ from their own" (APA, 1992, p. 1601). It is this reasoning that leads Throckmorton (1998) and Yarhouse (1998) to assert that it is unethical to force individuals who are unhappy with their same-sex attractions into accepting a lesbian, gay, or bisexual (LGB)-affirmative identity because it goes against the clients' religious choices, diversity, and moral convictions. They argue that an "out" LGB-affirmative identity may prove too difficult for some individuals insofar as it presents a constricted range of choices that are unacceptable alternatives to leaving spouse, children, church, and community. Literature exists to support the idea that therapy can have a better outcome when therapists utilize counseling interventions that respect the principal values and goals of clients' religion (Bergin, 1980; Worthington, 1988). For example, Koltko (1990) provided an analysis of how religious beliefs affect psychotherapy:

Religious beliefs help to form a client's attitudes about the self and its worth, about what that self should become, and provide answers to questions such as: What forms of lifestyle are to be preferred? Which forms of human experience are pathological, which are merely normal, and which are genuinely and healthily transcendent? In brief, religious beliefs can influence every part of the personality. (p. 139)

In support of this position, McConaghy (1977) argued that individuals seeking conversion treatments should not be considered as victims of society but rather as capable of making a voluntary and knowledgeable request in accordance with their values and needs. Sturgis and Adams (1978) agreed and claimed that banning conversion therapy would indicate a failure to accurately assess and satisfy clients' needs.

On the other side of this debate are LGB-affirmative mental health organizations and therapists who argue that so-called non-gay clients do not have the freedom to be who they are, given the homophobic and heterosexist beliefs that pervade society. The underlying premise to treat homosexuality, as stated by Spitzer (1981), is a value judgment of whether "homosexuality and heterosexuality are essentially comparable conditions, differing only in prevalence" (p. 213). However, heterosexual bias, defined by Morin (1977) as a "belief system that values heterosexuality as superior to and/or more 'natural' than homosexuality" (p. 629), undeniably exists. This bias is known to foster hatred, discomfort, and fear of same-sex intimacy, love, and sexuality while promoting the more conventional, heterosexual ideal. Individuals may internalize these critical, external assessments, and uncomfortable or painful emotions may become activated when encountering homosexuality. Externally, societal institutions and systems often force individuals to dissociate and fragment their lives rather than helping them consolidate and accept the possibility of living with an "out" gay identity (Coleman, 1982; Herek, 1984; Ritter and O'Neill, 1989; Drescher, 1998b). Silverstein (1972) addressed these ideological effects and how they relate to issues of self-determination and sexual reorientation:

To grow up in a family where the word "homosexual" was whispered, to play in a playground and hear the words "faggot" and "queer," to go to church and hear of "sin" and then to college and hear of "illness," and finally to the counseling center that promises to "cure," is hardly to create an environment of freedom and voluntary choice. (p. 4)

Begelman (1975) insisted that the very existence of conversion therapy programs strengthens biases against homosexuality, while adding to the self-hatred of the clients seeking an alleged cure. Agreeing with these criticisms,

Davison (1978) urged clinicians to conduct comprehensive assessments of clients' social and political systems, thereby focusing "on the problems homosexuals (and others) have, rather than on the so-called problem of homosexuality" (p. 170).

Those who criticize sexual reorientation therapy also argue that changing one's sexual orientation is not possible and that attempting such a change may cause harm (Haldeman, 1991, 1994; LeVay, 1996; Martin, 1984; Murphy, 1992, 1997; Stein, 1996). Many have asked what exactly is the basis for conducting sexual reorientation therapy if homosexuality is no longer considered pathological or a mental disorder (Tozer and McClanahan, 1999). After presenting what he calls the "inadequate and questionable science" of conversion treatments, Haldeman (1991) pointed out that mental health providers who use such interventions "commit consumer fraud, as this damaging practice simply does not work" (pp. 150, 160).

In line with the latter reasoning, on August 14, 1997 the American Psychological Association passed that a resolution based on its ethics code, that affirmed six basic principles concerning treatments to alter sexual orientation. The resolution supported the "dissemination of accurate information about sexual orientation, and mental health, and appropriate interventions in order to counteract bias that is based in ignorance or unfounded beliefs about sexual orientation" (APA, 1998, p. 934). In essence, the resolution requires a full discussion by the therapist of the client's potential for happiness as a gay, lesbian, or bisexual individual and communication that no scientific evidence exists that conversion treatments work. The American Psychiatric Association (2000) elaborated on its earlier stance that homosexuality is not a mental illness and recommended that practitioners refrain from using sexual reorientation interventions until these treatment modalities are placed under empirical scrutiny to assess risks versus benefits and long-term outcomes. Other mental-health provider associations such as the American Medical Association, American Academy of Pediatrics, American Counseling Association, and the National Association of Social Workers have made similarly strong policy statements against sexual reorientation therapy.

THE "GAY IS BAD" AGENDA: "CHANGE IS POSSIBLE"

Despite current LGB-affirmative stances, individuals continue to seek out–and a subset of therapists continues to offer–sexual reorientation therapy. "Ex-gay" ministries became visible to the public's eye from July 13 to July 20, 1998 when a series of "ex-gay" advertisements appeared in national newspapers, including *The Los Angeles Times*, *The New York Times*, *USA Today*, *The Washington Post*, and *The Washington Times*. These full-page advertisements were sponsored by 18 religiously conservative organizations, including the Christian Coalition and the Family Research Council. The text of these advertisements included the messages that "the truth may hurt before it can heal, but change is possible" and "if you really love someone, you'll tell them the truth . . . that homosexuals can change" ("We're Standing," 1998, p. A11). Anne and John Paulk (Paulk, 1998) became a "poster couple" for the "ex-gay movement" when they appeared in these ads, testifying of their happy marriage, their freedom from a homosexual past, and the possibility that anyone could change her or his sexual orientation. Similarly, Exodus International, one of the largest ex-gay organizations, promoted the need for and effectiveness of conversion treatments:

> Exodus upholds heterosexuality as God's creative intent for humanity, and subsequently views homosexual expression as outside God's will. Exodus cites homosexual tendencies as one of many disorders that beset fallen humanity. Choosing to resolve these tendencies through homosexual behavior, taking on a homosexual identity, and involvement in the homosexual lifestyle is considered destructive, as it distorts God's intent for the individual and is thus sinful. Instead, Christ offers a healing alternative to those with homosexual tendencies. Exodus upholds redemption for the homosexual person as the process whereby sin's power is broken, and the individual is freed to know and experience true identity as discovered in Christ and His Church. That process entails the freedom to grow into heterosexuality. (Exodus International, n.d., para. 2-3)

Although many testify of the possibility of changing one's sexual orientation (e.g., Dallas, 1991; Nicolosi, Potts, and Byrd, 2000a, b; Socarides, 1995), no definitive statement exists explaining what clients, therapists, or researchers consider change to be in sexual reorientation outcome studies. Stein (1996) remarked that clients and therapists may have different goals in mind when using conversion principles, such as extinguishing homosexual fantasies or behaviors, replacing homosexual behaviors with heterosexual relationships, or altering the fundamental sexual orientation. Freund (1960) noted early on that the "major criterion of success appears to be a change in the sexual behaviour of the patient; a homosexual is regarded as cured when he [or she] gives up homosexual practices and succeeds in initiating heterosexual conduct" (p. 315). Other outcome goals may include learning to cope with the periodic intrusion of homosexual attractions, reducing behaviors and thoughts enough to live by one's religious and moral standards, or living with celibacy. Nicolosi (1991) proposed that reparative therapy

> . . . can do much to improve a man's way of relating to other men and to strengthen masculine identification. As a result of their treatment, many

men have been supported in their desired commitment to celibacy, while others have been able to progress to the goal of heterosexual marriage. (p. xviii)

Based on clinical experience, Birk (1980) noted that most individuals who identify as homosexual before treatment continue to have some homosexual feelings, fantasies, and interests after treatment. However, Yarhouse (1998) emphasized that same-sex attractions should be expected after treatment, similar to recovered drug abusers who still have "cravings" and experience residual effects. Regardless of the disputable analogy that homosexuality is similar to a drug addition, the lack of uniformity around outcome goals is lumped together and "change in sexual behavior or in the gender of one's primary partner may not indicate any change in underlying sexual desire at all" (Stein, 1996, p. 530).

Further adding to the ambiguity of whether a "cure" exists for homosexuality, self-reports of sexual reorientation have not been consistent with objective data. For example, Conrad and Wincze (1976) found that physiological arousal measurements did not support the positive reports of those who had participated in sexual reorientation behavioral therapy. Freund (1960) discovered, using data from phallometric assessments, that the descriptions of clients' successes of sexual reorientation were imprecise and involved contradictions with follow-up investigations, "which throws doubts on the diagnosis either before or after treatment" (p. 315). To date, no rigorous and definitive efficacy studies have been performed identifying what can be changed regarding sexual orientation, and the discussion of sexual reorientation therapy remains polarized.

"GAY IS NOT ME": EXPERIENCES OF THOSE WHO DESCRIBE THE BENEFITS OF CONVERSION THERAPY

To bring more understanding to this subject, this article's author (Beckstead, 1999) recorded and analyzed the perspectives of 20 individuals (2 women, 18 men) who had undergone counseling to change their homosexual orientation. Qualitative methods were used to develop a grounded theory (Glaser and Strauss, 1967) and theoretical framework that was based on participants' individual interviews, journal writings, and a focus-group discussion. These individuals were selected to participate in the study because they self-identified as proponents of sexual reorientation therapy and reported that they had become "exclusively heterosexual" or experienced other successful outcomes due to such treatments. This sample represented a subset of a larger research sample (5 women, 45 men) that included both the proponent sample and individuals who had underwent conversion treatments but self-identified with an "out" LGB identity and reported being harmed by or opposed to such therapy

(Beckstead, 2001). The two research samples could be identified as either "converted" or "nonconverted" to the ideology of conversion therapy. The research sample as a whole was limited to those individuals who were European-American and members of the Church of Jesus Christ of Latter-day Saints (LDS or Mormons).

According to LDS doctrine, the highest blessings are reserved for those who fulfill the moral obligations of the LDS church, and significant doctrines declare that homosexuality is not a part of God's plan (*Doctrine and Covenants*, 1981). That is, "everlasting joy" and "exaltation to Godhood" depend on a heterosexual family. The LDS church has in the last decade offered an acceptance of and leniency toward individuals who have same-sex attraction, as long as they do not "indulge" in the "perverted acts" of homosexual behavior (Oaks, 1995). Brzezinski (2000), in her research regarding same-sex attracted Mormons, articulated the "process and pain of identity development when faced with the disparity between same-sex orientation and religion" (p. iv). This strong religious climate affected the lives of the participants in this study as well, and their stories reflected their struggle. The present study, therefore, provided not only a description of the experiences of seeking sexual reorientation via therapy during a highly politicized debate, but it also supplied a unique analysis of the experiences of homosexual individuals who have a strong religious background. A summary of the results from this study follows to highlight participants' needs before treatment, how they met these needs via conversion therapy, and their agenda to let others know of the benefits of self-determination.

Disease Model: A Need for a "Cure"

All participants in the "converted" sample emphasized that their religious identities remained central to their core identity. As one participant, Robert, remarked:

> The thought of living a gay lifestyle . . . never crossed my mind. It was never an option to me. My upbringing in the church, my belief system, was so much a part of who I was. That's who I was. The sexual orientation was peripheral and if the sexual orientation was not in harmony, then something had to give and I decided, almost subconsciously at that point, that I was not going to be homosexual.

In addition to this "peripheral" positioning of their sexuality, every participant had distinct, negatively critical and polarized images of what it would mean for them to "be gay"–perceiving severe limitations of what their lives would be like if they were to consider themselves homosexual. They discussed how they developed these beliefs from personal experiences, stories from others who had lived "the gay lifestyle," and statistics about the dangerousness of being gay. Overall, their attitudes about the lives of gays, bisexuals, and lesbians were derived from a stereotypical view that to be gay would involve a life of promiscuity, distrust, cruising, disease, selfishness, loneliness, and emptiness. As stated by Matt, "Whatever discomfort I might feel trying to conform to a heterosexual lifestyle would be far more preferable [than living a gay lifestyle]. . . . The gay lifestyle could not promise commitment with the integrity and devotion that such commitment can foster." Russ also commented that "being gay" was not the optimal choice:

> I don't think it lends itself to the optimal development of a person whether that is mentally, socially, morally, [or] physically. There's a good deal greater health risk I think associated with the gay lifestyle, in terms of contracting diseases. I think that it's not optimal and therefore if you really pursue our own interest as a society, we wouldn't reward or condone it.

Many participants claimed that their homosexuality was equal to an internal "dis-ease," such as diabetes, bulimia, asthma, and cancer. For example, Shannon felt "afflicted" by his same-sex attractions and wished he did not have this "insidious, insidious, horrific, terrible, plague." He continued by saying:

> I wouldn't wish this on anybody. I would rather have cancer. That's how I look at it honestly. I have said this many times because cancer doesn't affect my eternal progression. . . . Theoretically, I can be cut off from my wife and be cut off from God. . . . So this is much worse than any kind of disease that I could ever have.

Another participant, Jason, who wrote books about the benefits of conversion therapy and used the pseudonym of Jason Park, also viewed being gay as spiritually, emotionally, and physically dangerous. In one book, he used inaccurate statistics that claim that "less than 2% of the gay population survives to age sixty-five" (Park, 1997, p. 131). Despite these strong, disapproving statements, participants also described experiencing a degree of pleasure or passion due to their same-sex attractions. Clint seemed to sum up these conflicting experiences by stating, "I see it as a sad lifestyle, although it has some elements that I find appealing. Is that an honest answer?"

Participants emphasized that the generally accepted concept of "internalized homophobia" was not the primary motive for not wanting to be gay. They indicated that the essential reason that compelled them to change their sexuality was a spiritual need to conform to what they felt to be true. For example, John insisted, "No, the pain was not inflicted by my religion's or by society's intolerance of homosexuality, but by my own soul's sense of dissonance; being gay did not bring harmony to me in my life." Like other participants, Rex provided examples of how he felt that "something seemed missing" in his life because of his homosexual actions. Doug, who no longer practiced the doctrines of the LDS church, emphasized that he believed his reason not to be gay came from an internal sense of what is right and wrong:

> The thing I think I need to drive home is that I had no external pressure to change. All of it had been long gone by the time I got involved in reparative therapy, and I did it because I wanted to. . . . [Being gay] just feels funny to me. It's not what I want, you know, and the standard gay Nazi response is "Well, this is internalized homophobia." Maybe, but maybe not, you know. That's a cop-out. But there is something deep that has nothing to do with religion, family, or anything else that if I just calm down, mellow out, there is something that just feels weird about me being gay. . . . There's something just weird internally to me about setting up a household with his-and-his towels.

With these self-concepts of being diseased, damned, and in need of change, all participants sought help from their religion.

Religion's Agendas and Responses

Although participants' church leaders tended to provide support, many participants discussed their frustration with the leaders' responses. Muriel, for example, pointed out, "Some just plain have no clue." Dan commented on his disappointment:

> One thing that was very difficult for me to understand was why my [church] leaders couldn't get any inspiration for me. I understood why I might not be able to get answers; I wasn't worthy to. But why not my leaders? These were spiritual men. Weren't there any answers?

Several participants stated that they were threatened by their church leaders to leave their gay relationships or be excommunicated. Shannon verbalized the treatment from his church officials in this manner: "I've learned that people want to beat you into submission, or emotionally even." Forrest related that his experience of going through a church disciplinary council left him distrustful of church leaders:

> I had previously asked for support from bishops in dealing with the pain and grief that I was going through associated with being gay and a member of the church. Three bishops and my stake president told me they

didn't want to hear about it. When I confessed my wrongdoing, they couldn't decide what the next course of action would be and they left me in limbo for about a month. That, combined with their breaking a confidence and other events, left me feeling extremely depressed and unwanted.

Discussing the meeting he had with an official in the LDS church, Robert said, "He told me that this millstone would soon be taken off my neck. Little did he know."

LGB-Affirmative Therapists' Agendas and Responses: "Gay is Good"

Participants turned to many forms of therapy to resolve their conflicts. Therapists who proposed that participants should "come out" and leave their religion were described as unable to understand the complexities of participants' dilemma. Jason's dialogue with his first counselor seems to articulate the frustrations expressed by all participants:

I tried to explain the conflict to her between religion, my personal values, [and my same-sex attractions] . . . and she just kind of said, "Well, I don't see what your problem is. Just pick one." She didn't seem much help. She just didn't quite get it.

Jacob provided an example of how his therapist unintentionally pointed out the losses that Jacob would have if he chose to identify and live his life as a gay man:

I went down in my mind this path of finding a lover, leaving my wife, and losing everything I loved, which was my wife and my family and my church and my God, my relationship with Him, and not finding any real happiness in that relationship in my mind because by that point I had known other people who had been in these relationships and they were fleeting.

Barnaby agreed, "I couldn't see leaving all that behind."

The Need for More Choices

Because of the high stakes involved of losing family, friends, community, religious support, and eventually "eternal exaltation," participants felt that "being gay" was not a valid choice for them and asked for more options than having to be "that way." For example, Barnaby stated:

> What I don't like is the idea that it's inevitable. That someone grows up and suddenly they are 12 years old and they see a guy and they like his butt, you know, and suddenly they are gay. I don't like that.

Ace, who was struggling to get out of a lesbian relationship during data collection, wrote about her conflicts with her options:

> It tears me in two. I don't believe I have a choice. I'm supposed to be the good little Mormon wife–being faithful and virtuous. But that's wrong–of course I have a choice (we always have choices, don't we?) and the choice I've been making for the past several months is not the choice that I should be making.

Participants adopted a variety of coping strategies to eliminate or cope with homosexual feelings. These strategies included (a) intrapsychic defense mechanisms; (b) sexual and relational solutions; (c) emotional coping; (d) hiding; (e) religious solutions; and (f) escape, release, and suicide. These strategies varied in their effectiveness but were unable to eradicate participants' attractions. Attempting suicide was seen as the only solution for 8 participants. Dan, for example, wrote, "I felt like I couldn't continue to live in such pain. My alternatives seemed to be either to end my life or to straighten my life out." Similar to other participants, Paul wanted to destroy the homosexual self he could not live with:

> I really felt that that guy was out of control and was being controlled by circumstances and his body, and I wanted to be controlled by a higher power. . . . I was majorly heading downhill and that's when I was contemplating getting rid of the guy I didn't like.

Sexual Reorientation Therapy: "The Last Option"

Participants' distress intensified around their sexual, religious, social, and spiritual conflicts and their coping strategies became more maladaptive until they hit what they described as an emotional "bottom" that compelled them to seek out a therapy that would resolve their conflicts. In addition to the emotional distress, 4 participants reported that they sought conversion treatments after they were convicted of public sexual activities. Richard described his motivation for therapy in this way:

> I entered therapy in a complete state of crisis. My life was out of control. I had put my family at severe risk of being torn apart, losing my marriage and my children. After 14 years, I could no longer manage the double life

of addict [sic] and churchgoing family man. I felt I had no choice but to enter therapy.

Kent wrote about the consequences that he experienced for being "totally out of control":

> Suddenly I saw a picture of my own marriage falling apart . . . if I stayed on the path I had started down again. It upset me, bad. I literally went and locked myself in the bathroom and covered my mouth while I sobbed for grief over what I had been doing again. . . . I really didn't know how to deal with this, and that's when I got involved with reparative therapy.

Converting to the Agenda of Reparative Therapists

For participants in this study, sexual reorientation therapy seemed to represent the best coping strategy to self-determine and find a solution that would be congruent with their religious and societal values. It was, as Jacob emphasized, a therapy that would "go the way [these participants] wanted to go." Accordingly, participants stated that sexual reorientation therapists and support groups accepted them as heterosexuals and provided causal theories and interventions to replace previously distressful self-concepts with more acceptable labels and skills. For example, participants described experiencing relief and hope after learning from reparative therapy principles that all heterosexuals have same-sex needs for emotional closeness and that participants did not have to eliminate these needs, only the sexualizing of these needs. Paul explained:

> I started getting some books. I think that's where I started getting major change for me. I was finally getting some literature that was helping me understand what I was dealing with. . . . Then I had something to pin some hopes on.

Because of these etiological theories, participants stated that they were able to connect their childhood neglect and gender inferiority to the cause of their homosexual feelings and behaviors. As Matthew wrote, conversion therapy "ended up identifying root causes of depression and feelings of inadequacy that gave rise to the same-sex attraction, or at least to its acute stages." Participants overall valued and were converted to these etiological theories that seemed to provide them with a reason "outside of them" of why they acted homosexual, rather than the belief that they were inherently or genetically homosexual. This seemed congruent with their need to believe that "being gay" was not a part of them.

Furthermore, with a religious belief in Satan's role to tempt these individuals continually with "amoral" thoughts, participants seemed assured that they did not have to feel distressed about being attracted to same-sex others, as Jason explained in his book:

> Temptation is not identity. Just because you are tempted by homosexual feelings, it does not mean you are a homosexual. Satan may continue to tempt you with things from your past, although you have left them behind. . . . Some men also try to compare sexual experiences with men with the sexual experiences they have had with their wives. This is an unfair and unnecessary comparison. Since illicit sex with a man is counterfeit love, Satan is anxious for it to be intense and seem fulfilling. But like illegal drugs, it produces an abnormal high that does not last. (Park, 1997, pp. 117, 185-186)

Given these reparative therapy and religious models, participants were not punished if they had behavioral and cognitive relapses but were treated as addicts who were in recovery and seeking treatment. This shift in identity from sinner to penitent seemed relieving to participants. Overall, their same-sex (emotional) attractions, which were once considered as "unnatural," became reframed for participants as universal, heterosexual, and nothing to eliminate.

Experiences of Success

Along with the positive outcomes of relief, hope, and acceptance, the overall therapeutic benefits described by the 20 participants in this sample were (a) developing secure, same-sex, emotional relationships; (b) increasing gender identity congruence; and (c) decreasing homosexual behaviors and thoughts. These positive experiences seemed to resolve their previously distressful emotions and identities of being (a) "lost and alone," (b) a "sissy or tomboy," and (c) a "fag, dyke, or pervert."

Universality (Yalom, 1985) seemed to be a curative factor for participants who developmentally had felt "lost and alone" and had the opportunity to participate in a conversion support group. One such group was Evergreen, a support group for same-sex attracted, LDS individuals that offered participants the assurance "that individuals can overcome homosexual behavior and can diminish same-sex attraction and is committed to assisting individuals who wish to do so" (Evergreen International, n.d., para. 1). At the time of data collection, 9 participants were members of Evergreen and 16 of the 20 had been involved in such activities. These groups were described by Jason as "a nonsexual 'gay' community" (Park, 1997, p. 80) and were for many the most important part of therapy. Jim expressed the essential nature of his support group in fulfilling his emotional distress:

Evergreen was extremely helpful, but not with what we proposed it to do. Therapy is interesting for the theories it proposes, but the help I got from Evergreen has been the associations and friendships I've made. I've talked with 200 men, 50 intimately. That has been helpful. Therapy and counseling and all that–I wish I had the money back.

Shannon captured the overall feel of Evergreen with these words: "You're not bad, I love you, let's progress together." Overall, participants described benefits of receiving validation, normalization, added resources of information and accountability, and opportunities to be authentic and develop relational styles.

Participants described their treatments as focusing on feelings, labels, and behaviors of growing up a "sissy or tomboy," because of their therapists' belief that a gender-identity deficit was the "cause" of homosexuality. For the male participants, a program of learning and playing sports was incorporated into their treatment. Doug explained this process as an "emotional transformation" and an "identity change." Muriel also described a maturing into her true gender identity through therapy:

> I am a very active dreamer at night. . . . In my relationship dreams, I wasn't always the same gender. Sometimes I was a boy with a girlfriend, sometimes a girl with a girlfriend, and sometimes a girl with a boyfriend and sometimes I wasn't even sure what gender I was or who I was. This would really distress me in the morning and I would feel confused and upset throughout the day. . . . But I have noticed in the past year that I don't dream of myself as the guy anymore. . . . Perhaps my true identity is becoming more instilled inside me.

Overall, this focus on gender roles and gender-group membership seemed to develop for participants a new sense of belonging, self-efficacy, and acceptance.

In addition to these benefits, participants reported shifts in their previous identity of experiencing themselves as "fags, dykes, or perverts." These shifts seemed to occur because they reframed their sexual fantasies as emotional needs, learned strategies to manage their attractions by decreasing the frequency that they sexualized same-sex individual, and discontinued homosexual sexual behaviors through relapse-prevention techniques. Bruce, for instance, explained his process of coping with same-sex attractions:

> Ask yourself, "What is it you really want? Do you want to have sex? Do you want a friend? Where are you going with this? . . . I realized that my perspective was changing a little bit where at first I would be walking across campus and I would see a good-looking guy and start sexualizing,

> to where I was like, "You know, I wonder if I could be his friend. I won-der if we could really be friends." And it just kind of changed my focus. . . . And again, it's still my choice if I want to sexualize it. Yes, I could still be aroused, but it's not necessarily what I want to do.

Another way participants seemed to cope with the dissonance of having same-sex attractions and not being gay was in making a distinction between *being* homosexual and *doing* homosexual. That is, a person only *is* lesbian, bi-sexual, or gay if she or he continues to *do* homosexual acts. The importance of the dichotomy of being and doing lies in the possibility that participants did not need to accept a homosexual label or orientation. As Jacob reasoned,

> How come someone who is living in a marriage relationship can have adulterous feelings and they're not labeled as adulterer: "You are an adulterer. You have adulterous feelings. You will always be an adul-terer." (Laughs). . . . I just couldn't accept those labels.

To embrace the idea that "gay is not me," participants needed to abstain from homosexual behaviors and fantasies, as Doug stated: "The only thing that de-fines the difference between homosexual and heterosexual is behavior. I mean, if I'm sitting next to my straight buddy, the only difference between him and me is behavior." LDS church leaders also distinguished between "being" and "doing" when considering the repentance of members. For example, a promi-nent LDS church official, Oaks (1995), asserted, "We should note that the words homosexual, lesbian, and gay are adjectives to describe particular thoughts, feelings, or behaviors. We should refrain from using these words as nouns to identify particular conditions or specific persons" (p. 9). Similarly, John, who married approximately five months after our interview, explained,

> My sexual orientation is heterosexual. I am not what I would say cured. I believe that any kind of addictive behavior creates patterns in the brain that take a long time to change, whether it's drinking or taking drugs or whatever. I had established a pattern. . . . I feel now like I'm a heterosex-ual who has not been [hetero]sexually active.

As an outcome of therapy, many participants reported that their "homosex-ual problems" had ceased to be an issue in their lives. Paul exemplified this with his comment: "It's so nice to be at peace. . . . I don't feel controlled by it, and I carry on other stuff in my life now." Achieving control over how to live their lives seemed to provide a sense of empowerment, as stated by Rex: "I came to understand that I have a choice as to how I behave. Before therapy, I was frightened. After therapy, I am confident and able to recognize my choices and choose according to what I feel is right." Participants referred to this increased self-understanding and self-acceptance as finding "wholeness" and congruence. For example, Jim described his progress as

> ... a maturing process of becoming more accepting of life, more accepting of who you are, and more powerful in your ability to get what you want, see what you want, have a clear vision, and achieve a certain calmness of who you are.

Participants reported, however, that their sense of peace and contentment did not indicate a change in sexual orientation but a change in self-acceptance, self-identity, focus, and behavioral patterns. *No substantial or generalized heterosexual arousal was reported, and participants were not able to modify their tendency to be attracted erotically to their same sex. Yet, these same participants continued to self-identify as heterosexual.* That is, as they became converted to the reparative therapy model that defined them as heterosexuals *and* as they decreased their homosexual behaviors, participants could label themselves "resolved" of their homosexuality. This treatment outcome seemed to involve attitudinal shifts in what identity they could apply to themselves and what they could do within that identity. Their self-concepts seemed to develop into more acceptable ones, congruent with their values and needs. Overall, a change in how to define sexual identity seemed to occur rather than a direct change in sexual orientation. If anything, participants in this study may have reoriented toward asexuality (i.e., an absence of fantasies for either sex) rather than toward heterosexuality (e.g., Storms, 1980).

Participants' Agenda: Sharing Their Stories
That Options Are Available

Many participants mentioned the importance of sharing their stories of success to provide hope for other "strugglers." For example, John expressed in an Evergreen conference, "For a long time I thought change was possible for others, but not for me. I now know that change is far more difficult than any discussion can define, but that it is possible, and it is a choice–the most difficult choice I have ever made." The need to let others know that more options exist than identifying as gay, bisexual, or lesbian, to have these options available to explore, and then have the right to choose which options to live were recurring themes as participants talked about their agendas for participating in the study. As Jacob stated, "I think there needs to be studies that show that reparative therapy works." Matthew wanted to share his "growth process . . . to give others hope for change in society that says change is neither possible nor desirable." Robert conveyed, "There is so much to the contrary that reparative therapy doesn't work or that, you know, it's a forced thing, that people are uptight or whatever. I want to increase the truth that change is available."

In an addition to their desires to share their successful experiences, participants expressed concern and even anger during their interviews because they
believed they were being silenced or oppressed by the mental health organizations' resolutions against sexual reorientation therapy. For example, Barnaby
related, "I think that is a form of abuse. I really do because you're denying
someone the opportunity to look at an option. . . . That is very oppressive."
Richard also expressed his feelings on this subject:

> I am angry at the gay culture that perpetuates the lie that no one can ever
> change and if someone is gay, then the only mentally healthy thing to do
> is indulge all sexual urges indiscriminately. I am angry with the psycho-
> logical professionals for adopting the gay agenda, perpetuating that lie,
> and abandoning men like me for whom change is by far the most emo-
> tionally healthy alternative.

Russ talked extensively about his opinions of the 1997 American Psychological Association resolution:

> I think their decisions are largely political, whether there are any good
> studies that address the real issues. It is so politically incorrect to do any
> research that may even suggest that homosexuality should be in some
> cases open to remediation. It's just so politically incorrect that very few
> people are willing to look honestly at the question. . . . Just like anything
> else, there are risks that the therapy might not have the desired outcome.
> There are no guarantees, and the fact that there are no guarantees have
> been skewed and twisted by the gay community, the gay agenda, to the
> point that the absence of guarantee makes an honest attempt at therapy
> suspect. . . . It's just ridiculous in my mind that that mental health agency
> has largely abrogated its responsibility when it comes to providing op-
> tions for people who seek to exercise their right to self-determination.

Doug also stated his concerns and reasons for participating in this research:

> My big fear is that politically the whole idea of change, the potential of
> change, the possibility of change, gets snuffed out for political reasons to
> that you can't even talk about it anymore. . . . The person at the end of the
> food chain gets forgotten and the question of what I want, and how I
> want, and when I want becomes irrelevant. So I guess I am here to stand
> up and be counted.

Jim stated his own need to investigate this subject: "There's not much science
in it at all, science has dropped out. It's become political . . . a push for a desired

outcome. My agenda is to advance the cause of science." In sum, Doug discussed the need of more research to "cure" homosexuality:

> Just because somebody that has asthma isn't evil that doesn't mean that you should start silencing any research . . . or any discussion or any possibility of curing or changing asthma. . . . Right now there's really not a cure for cancer. Is it unfair for a doctor to say, "We'll see what we can do or we'll look to see what we can find?"

The Danger in Hoping for a "Cure"

One reason for participants to hope for a "cure" may have come from their religious background and belief in miracles (e.g., "with God, nothing is impossible"). Former president of the LDS Church, Spencer W. Kimball (1969), testified that such change was possible:

> After consideration of the evil aspects, the ugliness and prevalence of the evil of homosexuality, the glorious thing to remember is that it is curable and forgivable. . . . It is forgivable if totally abandoned and if the repentance is sincere and absolute. Certainly it can be overcome, for there are numerous happy people who were once involved in its clutches and who have since completely transformed their lives. Therefore, to those who say that this practice or any other evil is incurable, I respond: "How can you say the door cannot be opened until your knuckles are bloody, till your head is bruised, till your muscles are sore? It can be done." (p. 82)

However, promising that God and sexual reorientation therapy "will set you free" from homosexuality was not congruent with the findings of this study, at least not in these simplistic terms. Participants discussed a more complex explanation for their changes and discussed needing to alter their initial hopes. For example, Bruce stated,

> I'll probably never be cured. . . . I believe that men are always attracted to men, you know, it may not be sexual attraction and make them aroused or something, but if I have good friendships and I can maintain those friendships in an emotional closeness that I need with men and have a wife and kids and a family, then I will be very satisfied, you know, and feel good about my life and then to me that will be success.

In Muriel's words, one can find both a sense of acceptance of her same-sex attractions as well as a hope of a "cure" for them:

I think if your goal is to totally change the way you feel, then you may be in for a lifetime battle. . . . I guess my therapy goal has been to gain light and truth . . . to know how to handle my feelings of same-sex attraction without getting overwhelmed and feeling hopeless. And I believe that in time–not by ignorance–like [my therapist] taught me, that when we know who we are, then we naturally become that. . . . And if there are parts of us that need to be "repaired," the Spirit will fix them.

The danger in the acknowledgment that a "cure" may be possible is that it may lead an individual into a "failure" mind set. Hopes of experiencing heterosexual attractions and eradicating homosexual attractions may turn into disappointments. One participant wrote, for instance: "The truth is that I'm really struggling again with the pornography thing, which is extremely discouraging to me at this point." This participant had mentioned several times earlier in his journal and to others that he was "cured" of his homosexuality but discussed later how he felt defeated because he was not attracted to women and continued to experience homosexual arousal. In addition, all participants described their "conversion" as a long-term process that was often painful. These long-term hopes for a "cure" or resolution, along with continued "relapses," may be misunderstood as so-called weaknesses of the individual rather than the ineffectiveness of treatments and what is possible to change. That is, individuals who attempt sexual reorientation and fail in experiencing themselves as heterosexual may believe (or their family and church members may believe) that they have not tried hard enough or were not motivated enough. Individuals may internalize their continual failures, and any lack of progress may contribute to self-loathing, lowered self-esteem, and hopelessness. Those clients for whom reparative therapy is not the answer may realize this far too late after their long, painful process gets drawn out.

CLINICAL, RESEARCH, AND POLITICAL IMPLICATIONS

A subset of same-sex attracted individuals exists who seem to get lost in the polarized debate regarding whether a homosexual can or should become heterosexual. Should same-sex attracted clients in conflict be placed in reparative therapy or provided with an LGB-affirmative stance? Which therapy modality would be more effective and ethical in providing these clients with a healthier and happier lifestyle? Participants in this study suggested that reparative therapy was necessary and effective for them because it provided more options. However, the "nonconverted" participants from the larger research sample (Beckstead, 2001) described many harms from such therapy. Ethically, it is important to develop theories, research, selection criteria, and interventions that will resolve the conflicts with which these individuals struggle. Overall, providing a space for these clients to explore their ambivalence, misinformation, and complex choices may be the most healing factor. Brzezinski (2000) suggested that this safe space provides clients with the sense of freedom to look at all the options before them regarding the integration of their sexuality into their interpersonal and cultural contexts. One may hope that all LGB-affirmative and reparative therapists would support clients in making their own choices about how to prioritize the dimensions of their lives. However, as participants in this study suggested, some counselors still work from an extreme and biased perspective. The following clinical issues seem essential until a broader based treatment plan is developed that allows clients to explore issues from a variety of perspectives.

How Results May Be Useful for LGB-Affirmative Therapists

Participants stated that they needed more workable alternatives than the ones to which LGB-affirmative therapists seemed to espouse. All participants stated that identifying as "gay" was not a valid option for them, because they were unable to deviate from their religious convictions, life circumstances, and values. Haldeman (1996) pointed out that therapists will more than likely be ineffective if they impose contrary value systems on their clients. In general, LGB-affirmative therapists may need to evaluate their heterophobic biases when helping their clients explore options, such as managing the difficult adaptation to a heterosexual lifestyle (Isay, 1998).

Many aspects of conversion therapy discussed as positive by participants may be incorporated into the work of LGB-affirmative therapists. The effective therapeutic variables suggested in this study were finding peace and reconciliation with the identities of being "lost and alone" and labeled a "fag, dyke, or pervert," and a "sissy or tomboy." Changing maladaptive defense strategies and forming secure and intimate relationships were also important therapy issues for these participants as they learned to manage their attractions. At least seven clinical issues were prominent for participants in their satisfaction with their social, spiritual, sexual, and gender identities. These salient issues may transfer to all types of therapies and include (a) working within clients' religious values and relational needs; (b) exploring a range of options and creating workable alternatives; (c) enhancing self-esteem, self-acceptance, and self-control; (d) breaking compulsive cycles and replacing ineffective coping mechanisms; (e) enhancing honesty, authenticity, and assertiveness within relationships; (f) increasing gender identity congruence; and (g) utilizing support groups to decrease the individual's sense of isolation. Above all, the goal for clinicians may be to facilitate positive self-identifications, regardless of sexual orientation (Morin, 1977).

How Results May Be Useful for Sexual Reorientation Therapists

Four clinical issues were highlighted, based on participants' perspectives, which could have an impact upon the work of sexual reorientation therapists. These issues include (a) being clear about therapeutic goals and outcome possibilities, (b) being clear about the limitations of sexual reorientation theories and interventions, (c) exploring the effects of homophobia and heterosexism internalized by and acting upon their same-sex attracted clients, and (d) exploring clients' rigid ways of defining self, gender, spirituality, homosexuality, heterosexuality, and relationships.

Many individuals entering reparative therapy may do so in the hope that such therapy will eradicate their attractions toward same-sex others and increase heterosexual attractions. As previously stated, a successful therapeutic outcome for participants was more complex than "leaving homosexuality." Clients seeking a status of "ex-gay" or heterosexual must be informed that they may always be susceptible to same-sex sexual desires and that their change process may entail a very long and sometimes painful process.

The limitations of reparative therapy theories and interventions involve making causal interpretations from studies that are correlational, not causal, to confirm their hypotheses about the etiology of homosexuality and how to "repair" it. An alternative hypothesis of their theories could be that a so-called gender-identity deficit develops from the child feeling separate from same-sex peers and adults and not being able to participate in important social developmental lessons *because* of her or his inherent homosexuality and attractions to peers. Hirschfeld (1914) suggested early on that the poor father-son relationship could result from "masculine" fathers not knowing how to relate to or what to do with a homosexual son's femininity or difference. In this "chicken or the egg" argument, reparative therapists ignore the possibility of alternative hypotheses by inferring the cause of sexual orientation using gender-identity data. Freund (1974) emphasized that a feminine gender identity was not a necessary condition for the development of male homosexuality, and *vice versa:* "The relationship between these two anomalies is either a relationship between their casual factors, or the presence of one of the two anomalies enhances the probability of the acquisition of the other" (p. 59). To test these hypotheses, Freund and Blanchard (1983) conducted three separate studies and found a consistent pattern of results that suggested that the emotionally distant relationships of fathers and gay sons relate to the sons' atypical childhood gender identity (or observed gender-role behavior) rather than to the sons' sexual attraction to males. Additionally, Storms (1980) tested whether a sex-role or erotic orientation determines sexual orientation. The results of Storms' study suggested that participants did not differ significantly on measures of masculinity and femininity; that is, sexual orientation did not necessarily involve sex roles but depended on sexual fantasies and desires. Furthermore, studies of non-clinical populations have failed to find associations between family patterns and the development of any particular sexual orientation (Siegelman, 1981; Bell, Weinberg, and Hammersmith, 1981).

As noted in this study, individuals who are trying to cope by seeking reasons for their homosexuality may tend to believe that reparative therapy hypotheses are proven facts. These leaps of causation may be misleading when participants who are seeking information have the possibility of being misinformed and believing that they are basing their judgments on science. Reparative therapists need to consider more sophisticated distinctions between sexual orientation, gender identity, and sexuality, and how these issues interact with attachment issues within relationships.

A consistent finding in this study was that participants held perceptions that were similar to reparative therapists that LGB relationships are "brief and very volatile, with much fighting, arguing, making-up again, and continual disappointments" (Nicolosi, 1991, p. 110). Participants stated they did not want to have these types of relationships and believed, as does Nicolosi, that gay relationships "almost never possess the mature elements of quiet consistency, trust, mutual dependency, and sexual fidelity characteristic of highly functioning heterosexual marriages" (p. 110). The stance of "gay is not me" seemed grounded in these pejorative stereotypes. This view is not consistent with well-established, empirical evidence that indicates that homosexuality *per se* is not an unhappy or unhealthy state of being (Gonsiorek, 1991) and that gay and lesbian relationships can be meaningful and stable (Peplau, 1993). In addition, the statistics that participants used to support their views of homosexuality as "dangerous" were referenced from studies by Cameron (1993), which have been discredited as fraudulent. Herek (1998), for example, detailed the statistical and validity errors of the Cameron group studies and noted their "substantial impact . . . to promote stigma and to foster unfounded stereotypes of lesbians and gay men as predatory, dangerous, and diseased" (p. 247). Ego-dystonic, same-sex attracted clients may forget that homosexuality does not represent a personality or lifestyle; it represents a sexual orientation (Morin, 1977). "Addictive" and "promiscuous" sexual behaviors may have unhealthy aspects, such as those experienced by some participants. However, it would be more accurate to remove the words "gay lifestyle" from one's terminology and use words such as compulsiveness, maladaptive coping, and substance abuse, in addition to issues of commitment and intimacy, with which all humans are faced, not just gay men, lesbians, and bisexual women or men.

As Murphy (1997) noted, "patients may unwittingly absorb the therapist's views on sexual orientation without due reflection" (p. 93). Therefore, biases that reflect issues of internalized homophobia and heterosexism must be explored between therapists and their clients within the sexual reorientation therapy setting. Therapists must also consider fully with clients the benefits and disadvantages of adapting to a range of heterosexual and homosexual lifestyles. To facilitate this exploration, introductions to role models of all perspectives may be helpful in dispelling stereotypes and empowering clients in their decision process.

Research Implications

Those conducting investigations into the efficacy of sexual reorientation must take into consideration the questionable reliability and self-presentational biases of surveys based on self-report (Leary, 1994; Schlenker and Weigold, 1992). Participants who identified as heterosexual in this study would more than likely have done so on surveys that ask similar questions regarding outcome change. Questionnaires that do not explore the meanings of participants' definitions of sexual orientations and reports of change may not only be meaningless due to oversimplification, but also misleading if they perpetuate an ideology that gays, lesbians, and bisexuals can and should be heterosexual. Individuals who are seeking a "cure" for themselves, family members, or friends may be susceptible to the imprecise messages of so-called ex-gays and of conversion therapists. Unbiased and objective data, such as psycho-physiological data from sexual arousal assessments, are needed to corroborate self-report findings and understand what type of change is possible in sexual reorientation.

Although participants in the present study expressed satisfaction with their experiences in conversion therapy, several repeated an important theme that more understanding and research are needed. In terms of defining the therapy, participants stated that even the name "reparative therapy" was problematic. One participant argued, "We are using the wrong words, asking the wrong questions, and approaching it so narrowly. . . . We've watched a lot of guys. It's not working. Now what else can we do?" Consequently, more empirical studies must be designed that examine the efficacy of both LGB-positive and conversion therapies. Researchers who investigate issues of sexual orientation are encouraged to be explicit about their values and distinguish their advocacy behaviors from their research behaviors.

Political Implications

Although it is important to recognize the legitimacy of the choices and self-defined successes made by participants in this study, this stance is not the same as condoning reparative therapy. As a result of conducting this study, it became apparent that some elements of conversion therapy are very effective at facilitating self-acceptance and self-identity, and some are not. The aspects of reparative therapy that work seem to be those components found in all meaningful therapy: providing normalization, support, reframing, workable solutions, and empowerment. The ineffective and harmful aspects of this therapy seem to be the misrepresentation of treatment outcomes, reinforcement of negative stereotypes, and internalization of treatment failure. Information is also needed regarding the spouses of those who marry "ex-gay" individuals. However, participants in this study indicated that LGB-affirmative therapy would not have been helpful for them. Therefore, working from a broader perspective may allow for accurate labels of sexual orientation without the added stigma, assumptions, or forced identifications. A treatment plan is necessary that is flexible and unbiased enough to help clients explore all options available, not one that pushes one agenda over another.

Overarching this finding is the author's belief that the bigger political and societal picture gets missed in the debate between reparative and LGB-affirmative therapists, as well as between ex-gays and gays. Religion also plays a role in this debate due to its imposed penalties and powerful influence to dictate members' attitudes and behaviors. These groups confront each other with divergent value systems, expect one another to conform, and then angrily disagree with any opposition. With this, the channels of communication, understanding, and connection get shut down. Recognition must be made between these groups that psychology may not be able to change the doctrines of religion and that religion may not be able to change the intentions of LGB-affirmative clinicians and researchers. Nevertheless, seeking dialogue toward a common ground that draws upon the strengths of each divergent viewpoint seems more productive than debating. In bridging this gap, changes can be made in the acceptance, honesty, and understanding of all groups and the creation of a forum for all voices to be heard and respected. Without this dialogue, these groups may miss the more important societal goal that it is not really about changing sexual orientation but ceasing the intolerance, discrimination, and separation that exist in society.

In summary, much variability exists in the way individuals adapt and live out their sexuality and spirituality in their social contexts. Rather than a polarization between a gay identity and a heterosexual identity and a need to label people as one way or the other, space must be created to embrace this variability and explore the many facets of our human identities. The ideal society for all seems to be a place where individuals can be "who they are" and be valued for it.

REFERENCES

American Psychiatric Association (2000), Commission on Psychotherapy by Psychiatrists (COPP): Position statement on therapies focused on attempts to change sexual orientation (Reparative or conversion therapies). *Amer. J. Psychiat.*, 157: 1719-1721.

American Psychological Association (1992), Ethical principles of psychologists and code of conduct. *Amer. Psychology*, 47:597-1611.

_____ (1998), Appropriate therapeutic responses to sexual orientation in the proceedings of the American Psychological Association, Incorporated, for legislative year 1997. *Amer. Psychologist*, 53:882-939.

Bayer, R. (1981), *Homosexuality in American Psychiatry: The Politics of Diagnosis.* New York: Basic Books.

Beckstead, A. L. (1999), "Gay is not me": Seeking congruence through sexual reorientation therapy. Unpublished master's thesis, University of Utah.

_____ (2001), The process toward self-acceptance and self-identity of individuals who underwent sexual reorientation therapy. Unpublished doctoral dissertation, University of Utah.

Begelman, D. A. (1975), Ethical and legal issues of behavior modification. In: *Progress in Behavior Modification*, ed. M. Hersen, R. Eisler & P. M. Miller. New York: Academic Press, pp. 159-189.

Bell, A. P., Weinberg, M. S. & Hammersmith, S. K. (1981), *Sexual Preference: Its Development in Men and Women.* Bloomington, IN: Indiana University Press.

Bergin, A. E. (1980), Psychotherapy and religious values. *J. Consult. Clin. Psychology*, 48:95-105.

Birk, L. (1980), The myth of classical homosexuality. Views of a behavioral psychotherapist. In: *Homosexual Behavior*, ed. J. Marmor. New York: Basic Books. pp. 376-390.

Brzezinski, L. G. (2000), Dealing with disparity: Identity development of same-sex attracted/gay men raised in the Church of Jesus Christ of Latter-day Saints. Unpublished doctoral dissertation, University of Utah.

Cameron, P. (1993), *Medical Consequences of What Homosexuals Do.* Washington, DC: Family Research Institute.

Coleman, E. (1982), Developmental stages of the coming-out process. *J. Homosexuality*, 7: 41-43.

Conrad, S. R. & Wincze, J. P. (1976), Orgasmic reconditioning: A controlled study of its effects upon the sexual arousal and behavior of adult male homosexuals. *Behavior Therapy*, 7:155-166.

Dallas, J. (1991), *Desires in Conflict: Answering the Struggle for Sexual Identity.* Eugene, OR: Harvest House.

Davison, G. C. (1978), Not can but ought: The treatment of homosexuality. *J. Consult. Clin. Psychology*, 46:170-172.

Doctrine and Covenants. (1981), Salt Lake City, Utah: The Church of Jesus Christ of Latter-day Saints (Original work published 1835).

Drescher, J. (1998a), I'm your handyman: A history of reparative therapies. *J. Homosexuality*, 36:19-42.

_____ (1998b), *Psychoanalytic Therapy and the Gay Man.* Hillsdale, NJ: The Analytic Press.

Evergreen International. (n.d.), *Evergreen International: Mission statement.* Salt Lake City, UT: Author. Retrieved April 12, 2001, from the World Wide Web: <http://www.evergreen-intl.org/Open.ivnu>.

Exodus International. (n.d.), *About Exodus: Policy on homosexuality.* Seattle, WA: Author. Retrieved April 12, 2001, from the World Wide Web: <http://www. exodusnorthamerica.org/aboutus/aboutdocs/a0000048.html>.

Freund, K. (1960), Some problems in the treatment of homosexuality. In: *Some Problems in the Treatment of Homosexuality,* ed. H. J. Eysenck. London: Pergamon Press, pp. 312-326.

_____ (1974), The phobic theory of male homosexuality. *Arch. Gen. Psychiat.,* 31:495-499.

_____ & Blanchard, R. (1983), Is the distant relationship of fathers and homosexual sons related to the sons' erotic preference for male partners, or to the sons' atypical gender identity, or to both? *J. Homosexuality,* 9:7-25.

Glaser, B. G. & Strauss, A. (1967), *The Discovery of Grounded Theory: Strategies for Qualitative Research.* Chicago: Aldine.

Gonsiorek, J. C. (1991), The empirical basis for the demise of the illness model of homosexuality. In: *Homosexuality: Research Implications for Public Policy,* ed. J. C. Gonsiorek & J. D. Weinrich. Newbury Park, CA: Sage, pp. 115-136.

Haldeman, D. C. (1991), Sexual orientation conversion therapy for gay men and lesbians: A scientific examination. In: *Homosexuality: Research Implications for Public Policy,* ed. J. C. Gonsiorek & J. D. Weinrich. Newbury Park, CA: Sage, pp. 149-160.

_____ (1994), The practice and ethics of sexual orientation conversion therapy. *J. Consult. Clin. Psychology,* 62:221-227.

_____ (1996), Spirituality and religion in the lives of lesbians and gay men. In: *Textbook of Homosexuality and Mental Health,* ed. R. P. Cabaj & T. S. Stein. Washington, DC: American Psychiatric Press, pp. 881-896.

Herek, G. (1984), Beyond homophobia: A social psychological perspective on attitudes toward lesbians and gay men. *J. Homosexuality,* 10:1-19.

_____ (1998), Bad science in the service of stigma: A critique of the Cameron group's survey studies. In: *Stigma and Sexual Orientation: Understanding Prejudice Against Lesbians, Gay Men, and Bisexuals. Psychological Perspectives on Lesbian and Gay Issues, Vol. 4,* ed. G. Herek. Thousand Oaks, CA: Sage, pp. 223-255.

Hirschfeld, M. (1914), *The Homosexuality of Men and Women,* trans. M. A. Lombardi-Nash. Amherst, NY: Prometheus Books.

Isay, R. I. (1998), Heterosexually married homosexual men: Clinical and developmental issues. *Amer. J. Orthopsychiat.,* 68:424-432.

Kimball, S. W. (1969), *The Miracle of Forgiveness.* Salt Lake City, UT: Bookcraft.

Koltko, M. E. (1990), How religious beliefs affect psychotherapy: The example of Mormonism. *Psychother.,* 27:132-141.

Leary, M. (1994), *Self-presentation: Impression Management and Interpersonal Behavior.* Pacific Grove, CA: Brooks/Cole.

LeVay, S. (1996), *Queer Science: The Use and Abuse of Research in Homosexuality.* Cambridge, MA: Massachusetts Institute of Technology Press.

Martin, A. (1984), The emperor's new clothes: Modern attempts to change sexual orientation. In: *Innovations in Psychotherapy with Homosexuals,* ed. T. Stein & E. Hetrick. Washington, DC: American Psychiatric Press, pp. 24-57.

McConaghy, N. (1977), Behavioral interventions in homosexuality. *J. Homosexuality*, 2:221-227.

Moberly, E. (1983), *Homosexuality: A New Christian Ethic*. Cambridge, England: James Clark.

Morin, S. F. (1977), Heterosexual bias in psychological research on lesbianism and male homosexuality. *Amer. Psychology*, 32:629-637.

Murphy, T. F. (1992), Redirecting sexual orientation: Techniques and justifications. *J. Sex Res.*, 29:501-523.

_____ (1997), *Gay Science: The Ethics of Sexual Orientation Research*. New York: Columbia University Press.

Nicolosi, J. (1991), *Reparative Therapy of Male Homosexuality*. Northvale, NJ: Jason Aronson.

_____ (1993), *Healing Homosexuality*. Northvale, NJ: Jason Aronson.

_____ Byrd, A. D. & Potts, R. W. (2000a), Beliefs and practices of therapists who practice sexual reorientation psychotherapy. *Psychological Rev.*, 86:689-702.

_____ (2000b), Retrospective self-reports of changes in homosexual orientation: A consumer survey of conversion therapy clients. *Psychological Rep.*, 86:1071-1088.

Oaks, D. H. (1995, October), Same-gender attraction. *Ensign*, 25:7-14.

Park, J. (1997), *Resolving Homosexual Problems: A Guide for LDS Men*. Salt Lake City, UT: Century.

Paulk, J. (1998), *Not Afraid to Change: The Remarkable Story of How One Man Overcame Homosexuality*. Mukilleo, WA: Winepress.

Peplau, L. A. (1993), Lesbian and gay relationships. In: *Psychological Perspectives on Lesbian and Gay Male Experiences*, ed. L. D. Garnets & D. C. Kimmel. New York: Columbia University Press, pp. 395-419.

Ritter, K. & O'Neill, C. (1989), Moving through loss: The spiritual journey of gay men and lesbian women. *J. Counsel. Develop.*, 68:9-14.

Schlenker, B. R. & Weigold, M. F. (1992), Interpersonal processes involving impression regulation and management. *Annual Rev. Psychology*, 43:133-168.

Siegel, E. (1988), *Female Homosexuality: Choice Without Volition*. Hillsdale, NJ: The Analytic Press.

Siegelman, M. (1981), Parental background of male homosexuals and heterosexuals: A cross-national replication. *Arch. Sexual Behavior*, 10:505-513.

Silverstein, C. (1972, October), Behavior modification and the gay community. Paper presented at annual meeting of the Association for the Advancement of Behavior Therapy, New York City.

Socarides, C. (1995), *Homosexuality: A Freedom Too Far. A Psychoanalyst Answers 1000 Questions About Causes and Cure and the Impact of the Gay Rights Movement on American Society*. Phoenix, AZ: Adam Margrave.

Spitzer, R. L. (1981), The diagnostic status of homosexuality in DSM-III: A reformulation of the issues. *Amer. J. of Psychiat.*, 138:210-215.

Stein, T. S. (1996), A critique of approaches to changing sexual orientation. In: *Textbook of Homosexuality and Mental Health*, ed. R. P. Cabaj & T. S. Stein. Washington, DC: American Psychiatric Press, pp. 525-537.

Storms, M. D. (1980), Theories of sexual orientation. *J. Personality Social Psychology*, 38: 783-792.

Sturgis, E. T. & Adams, H. E. (1978), The right to treatment: Issues in the treatment of homosexuality. *J. Consult. Clin. Psychology*, 46:165-169.

Throckmorton, W. (1998), Attempts to modify sexual orientation: A review of outcome literature and ethical issues. *J. Mental Health Counsel.*, 20:283-304.

Tozer, E. E. & McClanahan, M. K. (1999), Treating the purple menace: Ethical considerations of conversion therapy and affirmative alternatives. *Counsel. Psychologist*, 27:722-742.

We're standing for the truth that homosexuals can change. (1998, July 27), *Los Angeles Times*, p. A11.

Worthington, E. L. (1988), Understanding the values of religious clients: A model and its application to counseling. *J. Counsel. Psychology*, 35:166-174.

Yalom, I. D. (1985), *The Theory and Practice of Group Psychotherapy*. New York: Basic Books.

Yarhouse, M. (1998), When clients seek treatment for same-sex attraction: Ethical issues in the "right to choose" debate. *Psychother.*, 35:234-259.

Therapeutic Antidotes:
Helping Gay and Bisexual Men
Recover from Conversion Therapies

Douglas C. Haldeman, PhD

SUMMARY. Studies of sexual orientation conversion therapies have focused on the efficacy, or lack thereof, of treatments designed to change sexual orientation. Recently, given the typically low success rate achieved in most conversion therapy studies, some researchers have examined the potential for such treatments to harm patients. It is the author's impression, after twenty years' clinical work with individuals who have undergone some form of conversion therapy, that these treatments can indeed be harmful. This article identifies the various problems commonly presented by patients following an unsuccessful therapeutic attempt to change sexual orientation. Such problems include poor self-esteem and depression, social withdrawal, and sexual dysfunction. Case material illustrates these concerns, and therapeutic approaches to address them are suggested. Directions for future study are identified. *[Article copies available for a fee from The Haworth Document Delivery Service: 1-800-HAWORTH E-mail address: <getinfo@haworthpressinc.com> Website: <http://www. HaworthPress.com> © 2001 by The Haworth Press, Inc. All rights reserved.]*

KEYWORDS. Gay and bisexual men, homosexuality, conversion therapy, reparative therapy

Douglas C. Haldeman is affiliated with the University of Washington.

[Haworth co-indexing entry note]: "Therapeutic Antidotes: Helping Gay and Bisexual Men Recover from Conversion Therapies." Haldeman, Douglas C. Co-published simultaneously in *Journal of Gay & Lesbian Psychotherapy* (The Haworth Medical Press, an imprint of The Haworth Press, Inc.) Vol. 5, No. 3/4, 2001, pp. 117-130; and: *Sexual Conversion Therapy: Ethical, Clinical and Research Perspectives* (ed: Ariel Shidlo, Michael Schroeder, and Jack Drescher) The Haworth Medical Press, an imprint of The Haworth Press, Inc., 2001, pp. 117-130. Single or multiple copies of this article are available for a fee from The Haworth Document Delivery Service [1-800-HAWORTH, 9:00 a.m. - 5:00 p.m. (EST). E-mail address: getinfo@haworthpressinc.com].

To date, the controversy over conversion therapies has focused almost exclusively on the question of whether or not they are effective. Only recently has the potential harm to patients of such treatments been considered (Shidlo and Schroeder, 1999). It is the author's impression, after twenty years' clinical work with individuals who have undergone some form of conversion therapy, that these treatments can indeed be harmful. The present discussion will consider common negative psychological *sequelae* of conversion therapies and suggest therapeutic remedies.

In 1998, the American Psychiatric Association adopted a resolution rejecting therapies based upon the premise that homosexuality is a mental disorder (American Psychiatric Association, 2000). This resolution notes that treatment for homosexuality is most often provided to people who have been adversely affected in some way by their culture or society, and that such treatments put some people at risk for a variety of emotional problems. The American Psychological Association (1998) adopted a policy on conversion therapy in 1997, which reaffirms the view that homosexuality is not a treatable mental illness. The resolution further opposes portrayals of lesbians, gay and bisexual men as mentally ill due to their sexual orientation, and reminds the practitioner of the numerous ethical principles related to the treatment of sexual orientation.

In addition, the American Psychological Association recently adopted practice guidelines for practitioners working with lesbian, gay and bisexual clients (American Psychological Association, 2000). One guideline in particular, "Psychologists strive to understand how inaccurate or prejudicial views of homosexuality or bisexuality may affect the client's presentation in treatment and the therapeutic process," offers empirically based suggestions for how a therapist might deal with a client whose discomfort with his/her sexual orientation is so severe that he or she wishes to change it. The policies of these professional associations support the rights of lesbian, gay and bisexual psychotherapy clients to respectful treatment that is not based on the disproved theory that homosexuality is a treatable disorder. Although these policies allude to the possibility that some patients will be harmed by attempts to convert their sexual orientation, they do not specify the nature of the potential concerns. The following discussion will therefore examine the issues commonly faced by individuals who have had adverse experiences in conversion therapy.

THE POTENTIAL HARMS OF CONVERSION THERAPY

The professional literature has examined the theoretical and empirical bases of conversion therapy (Drescher, 1998; Haldeman, 1994; Stein, 1996; Tozer and McClanahan, 1999). Theoretical discussions in the conversion therapy literature have included speculations as to what might cause a homosexual orientation, inevitably with the underlying assumption being that homosexuality is pathological. Usually, some variant of the "distant or absent father and over-intimate mother" configuration is blamed for causing men to become gay.[1] Such studies generally examine outcomes after a conversion treatment proce-dure of one sort or another; these have historically included behavioral (in-cluding aversive therapy), cognitive and psychodynamic interventions. These studies are characterized by serious methodological flaws that render them dif-ficult to interpret, and make it impossible to generalize from them. The most common flaws include subject selection and classification, defining what con-stitutes change of sexual orientation, the effects of response bias in self-report, and what follow-up is conducted to assess the stability of treatment effects. These methodological problems have been noted and assessed by several re-viewers (Haldeman, 1994; Stein, 1996; Tozer and McClanahan, 1999).

Even the most enthusiastic of conversion therapists claim roughly a 30% "success" rate (Haldeman, 1999). This low frequency is typically explained by the fact that sexual orientation is very difficult to change. Where others might consider a 30% success rate as less than optimal, in the domain of conversion therapy it is the accepted standard. The apparent lack of concern on the part of conversion therapists regarding their treatment "failures" is significant. Only recently, for example, has the obvious question been raised, "What about the other 70%?" (Shidlo and Schroeder, 1999). Given the tremendous psychologi-cal implications of trying to change something as profound and complex as sexual orientation, it might be reasonable to wonder if any harm results in the vast majority of individuals who do not successfully change in these treat-ments. That possibility has not been addressed, and is even ignored by conver-sion therapists who, because of a strong anti-gay bias, see any chance at changing unwanted homosexual or bisexual orientation as being worth what-ever risks might be involved.

What follows are the author's impressions of those risks, based on twenty years of clinical practice with individuals who have been through a variety of efforts to change their sexual orientation. Typical adverse responses have been thematically grouped according to the clinical issues most often presented by the treatment failures of conversion therapies. It should be noted that although these observations are not systematically derived, they do convey common clinical presentations of individuals who feel they have been harmed by con-version therapies. Clearly, all of the potential outcomes of conversion therapy need to be further documented and assessed.

The term "reparative therapy" has often been used interchangeably with conversion therapy. The term "reparative therapy," however, supports an inac-curate theoretical construct, namely, that homosexuality and bisexuality are a form of "brokenness." Therefore, the term "conversion therapy" is used here. It should be further noted that there is no universal response to the experience of having undergone a conversion therapy. Individuals' reactions may depend upon a variety of factors: their own constitutional resilience, the level of "invasiveness" of the treatment they have undergone, and the relative degree of social support, or lack thereof, that they enjoy. Not all individuals appear to be harmed by conversion therapy. It is not uncommon, in fact, for some to report that a failed attempt at conversion therapy had an odd, indirectly beneficial effect. This effect can be described as an individual's final "letting go" of the denial surrounding his sexual orientation. One patient stated, in reference to his experience in an ex-gay Christian counseling group, "I finally 'got' it. There was nothing else I could do and nowhere else to turn, so I figured I'd better get on with my life as a gay man."

Unfortunately, this is not everyone's experience. For many, a failed attempt—or a series of failed attempts—at conversion therapy signals an ending, not a beginning. The hope of conforming to social expectations of family, culture and church comes to an end with a failed attempt to change sexual orientation. With the end of this hope comes a host of potential losses: expulsion from family, loss of position in society, rejection from familiar institutions, loss of opportunities to raise children, loss of faith and community, and vulnerability to anti-gay prejudice. Combined with the difficulty that many "ex-ex-gay" individuals have integrating themselves into the gay community, the period following "unsuccessful" conversion therapy can be fraught with emotional issues. Generally, these include depression and guilt related to multiple losses, intimacy avoidance, sexual dysfunction, and religious and spiritual concerns. These issues can be overlapping in nature, and an individual may experience one, several, or all of them. They will be described in greater detail with brief case material, followed by suggestions for how therapists can address them clinically.

DEPRESSION RELATED TO LOSS

When asked why he attempted to change his sexual orientation—several times in individual therapy and in spiritually based prayer groups as well—Dan answered: "I just felt it wasn't *me* to be gay." When pressed further, he explained that he saw nothing wrong for others to be gay, but that it was incongruent with a picture he had of himself that included having a wife and children. Elaborating on this picture, he described a life in which he enjoyed support from his family and church community as a heterosexual, married man with children. Now, having been unable to make this fantasy a reality, he reported feeling very depressed, guilty and hopeless. He feared that the dream of support from his family would never come true if he were to live openly as a gay man; furthermore, he believed that he would no longer be able to participate in the church community that had been the mainstay of his social world since early childhood.

Conversion therapy alone did not induce Dan's depression. Rather, the failure of the treatment signaled to the client what he likely felt all along: that the social benefits derived from his family and community would require him to engage in a lifelong masquerade to hide his homosexual orientation. The fact that Dan now realizes the impossibility of this situation, however, makes it no less painful to relinquish. His future, which was once founded on a desired image of himself that would become possible with a successful course of conversion therapy, is now in doubt. He is letting go of the fantasy that he would somehow overcome a significant element in his identity in order to take his place in society, but as yet has nothing with which to replace it. He has no sense of connection to the gay community; on the contrary, he is afraid of what he perceives as its strangeness, and has difficulty conceptualizing himself as part of it. In general, he is plagued by guilt, and his self-esteem is contaminated with feelings of failure.

These significant losses require grief work. The feelings associated with these losses cannot be dispelled with optimistic encouragement to come out, be proud, find a partner and adapt to life in the gay community. Dan's first task is to acknowledge the pain associated with the losses he has suffered, and to begin neutralizing the toxic effects of the shame and guilt he has internalized. In so doing, he begins the process of disengaging what he will come to experience as his true self from the numerous expectations that have been placed on him. Part of the neutralization of shame takes place by examining a self that has been firmly embedded in a sociocultural environment that did not value the self for who it was, but that required it to change (or hide) in order to be acceptable. Ultimately this is not a problem of the self, but of the social environment. The environment, imbued with such powerful attributes as love, acceptance and potential for success, and the threat of eternal damnation, seemed implacable. Ultimately, however, one lesson of a failed conversion treatment is that life must be lived for the self, not for the environment.

In further assessing a depression related to loss, it is important to inquire specifically about what the client has learned about sexual orientation in conversion therapy. It is not uncommon for clients to need re-education, because conversion therapists have either convinced them that homosexuality is a state of arrested psychological development or a moral insufficiency. Initial research in this area (Shidlo and Schroeder, 1999) suggests that many clients in conversion therapy report that their therapists presented them with distorted information about homosexuality. This misinformation can only serve to intensify whatever guilt the client is already feeling. If there are inaccurate beliefs about sexual orientation that linger, they need to be examined and challenged. Shidlo and Schroeder (1999) also note that a significant number of conversion therapy clients report having lied to their therapists in order to please them. It is important to reinforce the notion that post-conversion therapy treatment does not require the client to switch to a pro-gay perspective. Although he will probably be experiencing ambivalence about his sexual identity, the ambivalence need not be hidden to please the gay-affirmative therapist. It should be treated as a welcome element in the treatment.

Gonsiorek and Rudolph (1991) propose a model of gay identity development that is useful in working with men who have just come out. This model is particularly useful for individuals who have recently abandoned conversion therapy, but as yet have a limited frame of reference for what it might mean, both psychologically and socially, to be gay. The model draws parallels with Kohut's self-psychology theories of childhood psychosocial development. According to Gonsiorek and Rudolph, the first stage of gay identity development involves an exploration of one's own narcissism. The gay man seeks encouragement simply to "be" himself, and as he is ready, avails himself of environments that provide support, encouragement and connection. Often, those who have struggled with conversion therapy have avoided the company of other gay men, save for impersonal sexual encounters. When the time is right, clients who are in the first stages of distress over identity disruption can benefit from being in the company of others who can reflect the new (gay) aspect of identity in a positive way.

An important concern with clients like Dan involves the individual's emotional state. It is important not to minimize the impact that the multiple losses of family and self-concept can have; some clients experience depression to the point of feeling suicidal. Suicidal clients should be offered the resources needed to keep them safe–including psychiatric consultation or hospitalization, if necessary. For more stable clients, it is important, in a gentle way, to offer resources through which the individual can inform him or herself about sexual orientation. In addition to a number of excellent self-help and workbooks available for newly out individuals (Alexander, 1997; Clark, 1997; Hardin, 1999; Signorile, 1996) there are resources on the Internet and support groups that meet in most medium-sized cities. In some cases, the treatment with clients such as Dan may amount to ego reconstruction.

INTIMACY AVOIDANCE

Intimacy issues are often of central importance in psychotherapy with gay men (Alexander, 1997; Haldeman, 2001). This can be especially true for clients who have undergone conversion therapy. Paul came to therapy following a lengthy, traditional "talk-therapy" format of conversion treatment that relied heavily on cognitive-behavioral interventions. Part of this therapy involved exercises in assertive behavior toward women and heterosexual dating. Paul reported that he realized, after many unsuccessful attempts at heterosexual relating, that he was "undeniably gay" and terminated treatment. In the time that followed, he believed that he had resolved all of the shame and self-recrimination he had experienced about being gay. However, he reported a pattern of difficulty in developing long-term relationships, which he attributed to a pattern of seeking out either unavailable or unsuitable people. Paul did not, however, connect this pattern to his experiences in conversion therapy.

Therapy with Paul revealed that his primary beliefs about himself as a gay man were not as settled as he had thought. Although he generally endorsed the belief that as a gay man he was entitled to satisfying, functional interpersonal relationships, he acknowledged that he still harbored a certain degree of critical judgment against himself for being gay. In theory, Paul reported, it was acceptable to be gay, but coming out tapped into a significant level of his internalized homophobia. This resulted in a pattern of seeking out unavailable men, or focusing on men to whom he was not particularly attracted, and then quickly losing interest in the relationship.[2]

The pattern of sequential, unstable attachments in same-sex relationships appears to be rooted in Paul's lack of acceptance of himself as a gay man. This lack of acceptance, and the implications thereof, need to be examined and understood before Paul will be able to participate fully in a primary relationship with another man. Furthermore, the adverse effects of Paul's conversion therapy experiences need to be understood. His efforts at heterosexual dating stemmed from a neurotic need to please his therapist, as well as his having adopted the belief that his value as a man was rooted in his success at dating women. The conversion therapy, which used the transference as the fulcrum on which heterosexual orientation ultimately develops, is responsible for Paul's intimacy dysfunction. Instead of achieving a heterosexual shift, Paul became doubly shamed at his gayness, as well as his failure at becoming a "real" man because of his inability to date women.

Conversion therapies typically rely on the therapeutic relationship to catalyze a shift in sexual orientation. The client is expected to identify with the male therapist, to bond with him emotionally, and to delight in his approval when the client is able to develop heterosexual relationships. When the process fails, the potential for harm is significant. The failure at heterosexual dating, once admitted, did not leave Paul an enthusiastic and self-affirming gay man. Rather, the awkwardness he felt in response to his failed attempts at heterosexual dating has been resurrected in his life as a gay man. Paul's homoerotic feelings trigger conflict between his natural arousal and the conversion therapy-induced overlay of shame. To correct this, appropriate risk-taking and careful exploration of the feelings associated with intimacy with another man set Paul on a path of interpersonal relating that was right for him.

Paul's case illustrates the second stage of Gonsiorek and Rudolph's model of gay identity development. In this stage, the individual has progressed through the narcissistic stage and is ready to internalize the values and beliefs of the (gay) community around him. Such values and beliefs that might be applicable to Paul have to do with the understanding that gay identity can be expressed in relationships, both affiliative and romantic, and that both kinds of relationships are positive and necessary enhancements for a fulfilling life.

SEXUAL DYSFUNCTION

Jim came to therapy having undergone one of the more brutal and psychologically invasive forms of conversion therapy: electric shock treatments. While still in college, Jim had agreed to aversive treatment for homosexuality on the advice of a leader in his church. This leader explained to Jim that unless he eradicated his homosexuality, not only he, but his entire family would be barred from heaven. A devoted son and brother, these words had such a strong impact on Jim that he agreed to undergo this treatment. As part of his therapy, he was instructed to visit pornographic bookshops and select homoerotic material that he found particularly arousing. During treatment sessions, Jim would view the pictures while an electric shock was simultaneously delivered to his hands and genitals. The cessation of the shock would be accompanied by heteroerotic material. The goal of this method was to extinguish homoerotic responses, and replace them with heteroerotic ones.

This treatment was not successful in changing Jim's sexual orientation. It did, however, leave him extremely confused and conflicted about his natural homoerotic feelings. When the conversion therapy failed, Jim finally acknowledged his homosexuality to his family who promptly disowned him. He moved to a large city, where he worked as a model. He tried unsuccessfully, with a number of individuals, to establish a loving relationship, but was troubled by chronic erectile dysfunction. These were the days before Viagra, and Jim was rarely able to sustain an erection. For him, sexual arousal was associated with an aversive experience. Additionally, he had deeply rooted shame related to his sexual response, partly as a result of his culture, and partly having been reinforced by his conversion therapy. His newfound cognitive recognition that it was permissible for to love another man paled in contrast to the firmly established sense of shame about his gayness, reinforced by conversion therapy. As a result, his new relationships were invariably affected by impotence. As the problem progressed, Jim started avoiding sex altogether.

Jim's situation is not uncommon among survivors of conversion therapies, although those who have been through aversive treatments seem to be especially vulnerable to sexual dysfunction. This may be due to the fact that aversive treatments affect the individual on a physical as well as a mental level, and the body responds in kind by manifesting ambivalence about sexual expression. The stress associated with sexual difficulties is often exacerbated by the sometimes hypersexual climate of the gay male community. Frequently, conversion therapy refugees who struggle with sexual concerns avoid potentially romantic or sexual situations and become socially isolated.

Sex therapy resources for practitioners working with gay men are somewhat limited, since most of the sex therapy literature is written by and for heterosexuals. However, work with clients whose sexual functioning concerns are in part attributable to a conversion therapy history is aided by the use of exercises that are equally applicable to gay, bisexual or heterosexual men (cf. Zilbergeld, 1994). These exercises vary depending upon the condition to be addressed. Typically, the sexual concerns of gay men who have been in conversion treatments include arousal problems or ejaculatory competence. The former can be successfully treated with sensate focus and relaxation exercises. The latter are often treated with the use of autoerotic exercises that gradually involve the introduction and participation of the partner. This assumes, of course, that a partner is available for practice, which is often not the case. Sexual concerns are partly caused by sex-negative attitudes, reoccurrence of the problem, and shame. Successful treatment of psychogenic sexual dysfunction requires that the attitudes and feelings surrounding sexual interaction be considered.

DE-MASCULINIZATION

Many conversion therapy models conceptualize homosexuality as an arrest in normative psychosexual development due, in part, to an inadequate identification with the same-sex parent. In order to correct this hypothetical defect, conversion therapists often rely on therapeutic transference to replicate the paternal attachment. Additionally, some conversion therapists encourage their clients to engage in a variety of "male bonding" activities, including attending and participating in sporting events, or visiting social venues for heterosexual men. In these conversion therapies, the desired shift to heterosexuality is strongly connected to stereotypically male social activities. For those who discontinue their conversion therapy, there can be an accompanying sense of lost masculinity. The client equates his failure at heterosexuality with failed manhood.

For a gay man, a sense of male identity is important, given that his affiliative and romantic relationships will be with other men (Haldeman, 2001). Some men feel de-masculinized after abandoning conversion therapy. This, in turn, has an adverse effect on self-concept and relationships with other men. Post-conversion therapy treatment often includes an assessment of the degree to which the individual's sense of "maleness" is intact. This means reinforcing the legitimacy of their decision to abandon conversion therapy. Furthermore, it may mean supporting them in developing a male identity consistent with their own sense of self. For some, this may still mean playing basketball, going fishing, or watching the Super Bowl. Conversely, it may mean engaging in stereotypically female pursuits, and yet not feeling less masculine. One's gender identity is the unique right and responsibility of the individual to define. It may rely upon conformity to stereotypical gender roles only to the extent that this matters to the individual.

SPIRITUALITY AND RELIGION

Without question, the single most difficult area to be navigated with many clients following conversion therapy is that of spirituality and religion. This is in part due to the fact that deeply held religious and spiritual beliefs can be as important an aspect of the self as sexual orientation. The reasons for this importance may be varied and complicated, but many individuals' religious beliefs and experience serve as a primary rudder in an otherwise anxiety-provoking, amorphous existence. Religion can be associated with comfort, structure, and the nurturing of family. As mentioned before, these are significant losses to contemplate. When religion and sexuality are in conflict, a tremendous obstacle to integration of the self is created. For most individuals, the very reason they sought out conversion therapy in the first place is related to their religious beliefs. The failure of conversion treatment does not necessarily dissipate the strength of the religious feelings, or provide an easy mechanism for reconciling them with sexual orientation.

Bill came to therapy seeking to reconcile his religious beliefs with his sexual orientation. After a series of ex-gay ministry experiences, he began to entertain the notion that perhaps he was intended to be gay, and that he should adopt a more accepting attitude toward himself. As soon as he abandoned his efforts to become heterosexual, Bill reported feeling an enormous sense of relief, and a deep spiritual conviction that he had taken the correct path. At the same time, he found that it was difficult to integrate his spiritual self with others in the gay community. He remarked that the challenges associated with yet another "coming out" process, of being a gay man with strong religious beliefs, was surprisingly difficult. One main reason for this is that the influence of organized religion as an oppressive force in the lives of gay, lesbian and bisexual people is without institutional parallel. Many mainstream religious denominations still preach that homosexuality is a sin, or at least that celibacy is a prerequisite for welcoming lesbians and gay men in their congregations. Many denominations still forbid the ordination of openly gay or lesbian clergy. These prohibitions are frequently used by persons who seek to justify their prejudice against lesbian, gay and bisexual individuals. For this reason, many lesbian, gay and bisexual people see organized religion in a negative light.

Nonetheless, Bill pursued avenues within the gay community where he could be both openly gay and a person of faith. At present, there are a number of gay-specific congregations and houses of worship, as well as numerous mainstream denomination "reconciling congregations" that welcome lesbian, gay and bisexual people and affirm their spiritual needs. After having found a home in one such congregation, Bill was much better able to integrate these historically conflicted, but important, aspects of his self.

This illustrates the third and final stage of Gonsiorek and Rudolph's model of gay identity development. Following the establishment of an integrated self, including positive introjects from the community, the gay person enters the "idealized" sector. In this stage, the gay person is "one among many," whose sense of self is maximized by a connection to others. In this regard, significant others and the community itself serve a surrogate familial function, offering the individual a context for both comfort and contribution.

Not all internal conflicts between religion and sexuality end with a successful integration, however. Clients whose strongly held religious beliefs cannot be adapted to fit the emerging understanding of the (gay) self are those most likely to abandon gay-affirmative treatment and return to conversion therapy. For some, the power of familial rejection and religious condemnation, coupled with the possibility of a poor connection with the gay community, is simply too much to overcome. While the majority of lesbian and gay individuals who come from unaccepting religious backgrounds appear able to separate from their histories, and if need be, their families of origin, in a healthy way, this is not the case for all.

CONCLUSION

Public campaigns promoting conversion therapy harm gay, lesbian and bisexual people by distorting the truth about sexual orientation, and fueling prejudice (Haldeman, 1999; Kahn, 1998). The relationship between the religious political activists whose "purpose (is) to strike at the assumption that homosexuality is an immutable trait" (Hicks, 1999) and the groups promoting conversion treatments has been documented. The publicity surrounding "cures" of homosexuals is intended to influence public opinion that homosexuality can be changed, and that gay men and lesbians should not receive anti-discrimination protection in housing and employment, and that "sexual orientation" should be excluded as a category in legislation against hate crimes.[3] The offering of conversion therapists by antihomosexual religious conservatives is therefore a significant element in reinforcing social stigma against homosexuality.

In contrast to the social harms of conversion therapy, activists and professionals alike have paid less attention to the potential adverse consequences of conversion therapy to the individual. The present discussion is a cursory examination of issues common to individuals who have undergone some form of conversion therapy, and highlights those concerns that deserve further, systematic study. Each case is unique, and the cases mentioned here are intended to offer the clinician a perspective on the kinds of issues that are frequently presented by clients, as well as some considerations as to how they might be addressed therapeutically. The issues of depression and poor self-image, relationship and intimacy avoidance, sexuality and spirituality are certainly not exhaustive. Research in this area will undoubtedly expand and refine this list.

It is important, however, to document that conversion therapy practices can have adverse consequences–some very serious–on numerous individuals. These range in severity from poor self-esteem, to chronic unhappiness in relationships and up to suicide. This is not to suggest that all conversion therapies are harmful, or that the mental health professions should try to stop them. It must be remembered, however, that a client's request to change sexual orientation is fraught with socially driven implications. Such a request should not be met with reflexive agreement on the part of the therapist, but should be carefully questioned and examined.

As long as antihomosexual elements persist in our culture and our social institutions, there will be frightened, unhappy individuals seeking conversion therapy. The time has come for the research in this area to shift from the question, "Does it work?"–a question that has been answered many times. The more important research questions that are finally being addressed are, "Why did you attempt a conversion therapy in the first place?" "Did it help you?" should be accompanied by, "Did it hurt you?" (Shidlo and Schroeder, 1999). For years, critics of conversion therapy have maintained that these treatments do not change sexual orientation. For the sake of the clients who have been harmed, it is time to learn more about what the effects of conversion therapy truly are.

NOTES

1. The neglect of lesbians in the conversion literature suggests that they are of less concern to these theorists.
2. Paul's case raises another issue that has not been addressed in the conversion therapy literature. As part of their treatment, clients in conversion therapy are frequently

encouraged to date members of the opposite sex. What are the appropriate procedures for disclosure in this regard? What responsibilities does the conversion therapy client bear toward the opposite-sex partners who are serving as therapy homework? These issues are absent from the conversion therapy literature, yet the ex-girlfriends, ex-wives and children of such failed "experiments" constitute a significant element of the conversion therapy equation. Their needs, particularly when the relationships they thought were likely to last fail because of a partner's undisclosed homosexuality, deserve attention in this discussion.

3. Antigay forces call attempts to gain such protections the "special rights" argument.

REFERENCES

American Psychiatric Association. (2000). Commission on Psychotherapy by Psychiatrists (COPP): Position statement on therapies focused on attempts to change sexual orientation (Reparative or conversion therapies). *Amer. J. Psychiat.* 157:1719-1721.

American Psychological Association. (1998). Appropriate therapeutic responses to sexual orientation. In the proceedings of the American Psychological Association, Inc., for the legislative year 1997. *American Psychologist*, 53:882-939.

American Psychological Association. (2000). Guidelines for psychotherapy with lesbian, gay and bisexual client. *American Psychologist*, 55:1440-1451.

Clark, D. (1997). *Loving Someone Gay.* Berkeley, CA: Celestial Arts Press.

Drescher, J. (1998). I'm your handyman: A history of reparative therapies. *Journal of Homosexuality*, 36(1):19-42.

Gonsiorek, J.C. & Rudolph, J. (1991). Homosexual identity: Coming out and other developmental events. In J.C. Gonsiorek and J.D. Weinrich (Eds.), *Homosexuality: Research Implications for Public Policy*. Newbury Park, NJ: Sage, pp. 161-176.

Haldeman, D. (1994). The practice and ethics of sexual orientation conversion therapy. *Journal of Consulting and Clinical Psychology*, 62:221-227.

Haldeman, D. (1999). The pseudo-science of sexual orientation conversion therapy. *Angles*, 4:1-4.

Haldeman, D. (2001). Psychotherapy with gay and bisexual men. In G. Brooks & G. Good (Eds.), *The New Handbook of Psychotherapy and Counseling with Men*. San Francisco: Jossey-Bass, 796-815.

Hardin, K. (1999). *The Gay and Lesbian Self-Esteem Book: A Guide to Loving Ourselves*. Oakland, CA: New Harbinger Press.

Hicks, K. (1999). Reparative therapy: Whether parental attempts to change a child's sexual orientation can legally constitute child abuse. *American University Law Review*, 49:505-547.

Kahn, S. (1998). *Challenging the Ex-Gay Movement: An Information Packet*. Somerville, MA: Political Research Associates.

Shidlo, A. & Schroeder, M. (1999, August). *Conversion therapy: A consumers report*. Presentation at the annual convention of the American Psychological Association, Boston, MA.

Signorile, M. (1996). *Outing Yourself.* New York: Fireside Books.

Stein, T. (1996). A critique of approaches to changing sexual orientation. In R. Cabaj & T. Stein (Eds.), *Textbook of Homosexuality and Mental Health.* Washington, DC: American Psychiatric Press, pp. 525-537.

Tozer, E. & McClanahan, M. (1999). Treating the purple menace: Ethical considerations of conversion therapy and affirmative alternatives. *The Counseling Psychologist,* 27:722-742.

Zilbergeld, B. (1994). *The New Male Sexuality.* New York: Basic Books.

Ethical Issues
in Sexual Orientation Conversion Therapies:
An Empirical Study of Consumers

Michael Schroeder, PsyD
Ariel Shidlo, PhD

SUMMARY. This study uses interviews with 150 consumers of sexual orientation conversion therapies to identify critical incidents of poor practice and ethical violations. We found that some licensed conversion therapists may be practicing in a manner inconsistent with the APA Ethics Code, similar professional codes, and recent guidelines on treatment of lesbians and gay men. Areas of ethical violations identified include: informed consent, confidentiality, coercion, pre-termination counseling, and provision of referrals after treatment failure. *[Article copies available for a fee from The Haworth Document Delivery Service: 1-800-HAWORTH. E-mail address: <getinfo@haworthpressinc.com> Website: <http://www. HaworthPress.com> © 2001 by The Haworth Press, Inc. All rights reserved.]*

Michael Schroeder is in private practice, New York City.

Ariel Shidlo is Psychologist, Columbia Center for Lesbian, Gay, and Bisexual Health, Columbia-Presbyterian Medical Center.

Address correspondence to: Michael Schroeder and Ariel Shidlo, 420 West 24th Street, New York, NY 10011 (E-mail: mschro@aol.com and ashidlo@aol.com).

The authors wish to thank Jim Jasper for his invaluable editorial help with this article, Huso Yi, MA for his untiring help as their research assistant, and Michael Radkowsky, PsyD and Paula Solon, PhD for their help with interviewing.

This study was supported by a grant from the H. van Ameringen Foundation.

This study was conducted in association with the National Gay and Lesbian Task Force.

A version of this article was presented in August 2000 at the American Psychological Association in Washington, DC.

[Haworth co-indexing entry note]: "Ethical Issues in Sexual Orientation Conversion Therapies: An Empirical Study of Consumers." Schroeder, Michael, and Ariel Shidlo. Co-published simultaneously in *Journal of Gay & Lesbian Psychotherapy* (The Haworth Medical Press, an imprint of The Haworth Press, Inc.) Vol. 5, No. 3/4, 2001, pp. 131-166; and: *Sexual Conversion Therapy: Ethical, Clinical and Research Perspectives* (ed: Ariel Shidlo, Michael Schroeder, and Jack Drescher) The Haworth Medical Press, an imprint of The Haworth Press, Inc., 2001, pp. 131-166. Single or multiple copies of this article are available for a fee from The Haworth Document Delivery Service [1-800-HAWORTH, 9:00 a.m. - 5:00 p.m. (EST). E-mail address: getinfo@haworthpressinc.com].

KEYWORDS. Conversion therapy, reparative therapy, ethics, psychotherapy, gay and lesbian

How can we determine whether sexual orientation conversion therapy is ethical, in theory and in practice? Both opponents and proponents of conversion therapies have discussed its ethics (Davison, 1991; Drescher, 2001b; Haldeman, 1991, 1994, 2001; Silverstein,1977; Throckmorton,1998; Yarhouse, 1998). Critics of conversion therapies have four objections: they (a) are not efficacious; (b) purport to treat what is not a psychological disorder; (c) devalue the lives of lesbians and gay men and reinforce prejudice; and (d) cause harm (Haldeman, 1991, 1994, 2001; Davison, 1991; Drescher, 2001a,b; Isay, 1990, 1997; Schreier, 1998). These objections have been echoed by the American Psychiatric Association which has recently published a position statement that until there is rigorous scientific research to substantiate claims of cure, "ethical practitioners refrain from attempts to change individuals' sexual orientation, keeping in mind medical dictum to first, do no harm" (American Psychiatric Association, 2000). Similarly, the American Psychological Association (APA) adopted guidelines for psychotherapy with lesbian, gay and bisexual clients that remind psychologists of prohibitions against discriminatory practices, including "basing treatment on pathology-based views of homosexuality or bisexuality" (APA, 2000), and "a prohibition against the misrepresentation of scientific or clinical data (e.g., the unsubstantiated claim that sexual orientation can be changed)" (p. 1443).

Conversely, proponents of conversion therapies have focused on the ethics of withholding this intervention from patients who request it. Yarhouse (1998) has argued that based on his understanding of the APA Code of Ethics (1992), "clients should be seen as having the right to choose treatment for their experience of same-sex attraction" (p. 249). Similarly, Throckmorton (1998) has asked that the American Counseling Association and other mental health associations "not attempt to limit the choice of gays and lesbians who want to change" because of an obligation "to respect the dignity and wishes of all clients" (p. 301). Stern, interviewed in Nicolosi (1999a), has stressed the absolute value of the client choosing a therapy that is consistent with his goals. He says: "It should be a client's right, totally and completely, to choose a therapy which is consistent with his goals and values. Psychotherapy which limits a client's right to decide where and how he is suffering, *and how he wants to grow out of that suffering,* is untenable for both parties–the therapist and the patient [italics added]." This is an absolutist perspective that overlooks the fact that professional ethics and standards of practice sometimes do place restrictions on a therapist's responses to a client's goals. For example, if a client's goal were to feel less guilty about emotionally abusing his spouse, most therapists would agree that their professional ethics would prevent them from assisting the client in this manner.

There is a paucity of empirical data on the extent to which conversion therapists' clinical practices are consistent with the APA Code of Ethics (1992) and similar guidelines from other mental health associations. The sources of data used in existing discussions have been limited to accounts by conversion therapists of their clinical work (e.g., Nicolosi, 1991, 1993; Socarides, 1978) or first-hand anecdotal reports of failed conversion therapies (Duberman, 1991; Ford, 2001; Isay, 1990, 1997; Moor, 2001; White, 1994).

In order to create an empirical basis for further discussion of ethical issues in conversion therapies, the authors interviewed consumers of these clinical approaches and identified critical ethical incidents. These empirical data can help determine to what extent conversion therapies are consistent with the ethical, scientific, and practice directives of several professional associations:

- American Psychological Association's 1975 resolution stating that "homosexuality *per se* implies no impairment in judgment, stability, reliability, or general social or vocational capabilities" (Conger, 1975, p. 633);
- American Psychological Association's (1992) "Ethical Principles of Psychologists and Code of Conduct";[1]
- American Psychological Association's (1998) "Resolution on Appropriate Therapeutic Responses to Sexual Orientation";[2]
- American Psychological Association's (2000) "Guidelines for Psychotherapy with Lesbian, Gay, and Bisexual Clients";[3]
- American Psychiatric Association's (1998) "Position Statement on Psychiatric Treatment and Sexual Orientation";
- American Psychiatric Association's (2000) "COPP Position Statement on Therapies Focused on Attempts to Change Sexual Orientation (Reparative or Conversion Therapies)";[4]
- American Counseling Association's (1999) "Discrimination Based on Sexual Orientation: History of the American Counseling Association's Position";
- American Psychoanalytic Association's (2000) "Position on Reparative Therapy."

The material presented in this study derives from interviews with consumers of mental health clinicians licensed as psychologists, social workers, psychiatrists, marriage and family therapists, and counselors. The professional ethics document most frequently referred to in this paper is the American Psychological Association's (APA) Ethics Code (1992). Although we recognize that clinicians who are not APA members are not bound by APA codes, the similarity of the APA Ethics Code (1992) to the professional ethics codes of the American Psychiatric Association, National Association of Social Workers (1996), the American Association for Marriage and Family Therapy (1991) and the American Counseling Association (1995) is such that the APA Code can be used heuristically as a proxy document for the purpose of elucidating critical incidents. In the illustrations below, we do not identify the profession of the clinician because we do not intend this to be a study of inter-disciplinary differences in ethical behavior toward lesbian and gay patients (cf. Liddle, 1999; Stein, 1999). Our work is intended to provide a conceptual guide for future empirical research on professional ethics in conversion therapies.

METHOD

Methodological Issues

Because we know so little about the experiences of consumers of conversion therapies, a qualitative approach seemed appropriate for this exploratory stage of inquiry. In addition, ethical principles and their application in psychotherapy are not easily reduced into quantitative data because patient, clinician, and intervention contexts are essential to their adequate understanding. Our methodological approach is inspired by that of Flanagan's (1954) paper on the critical incident technique, Garnets, Hancock, Cochran, Goodchilds, and Peplau (1991) report on psychotherapy with lesbians and gay men, and Pope and Vetter's (1992) work on ethical dilemmas encountered by psychologists.

A brief mention of the limitations of this study is indicated. The data presented in this paper do not provide any information on the incidence and the prevalence of ethical violations in conversion therapy. This exploratory study was based on the retrospective accounts of consumers. Their self-report may not always accurately reflect therapist behavior. Rhodes, Hill, Thompson and Elliot (1994), on a study of misunderstandings in psychotherapy, have written of the limitations of using retrospective data from clients: "Informants may . . . [engage] in narrative smoothing, that is, the process of changing a story when recalling events. Clients' retrospective reports that recollect misunderstanding events from the vantage point of distance may lose the detail of the event as clients make sense of the events over time" (p. 481). Complementary research needed would include interviews with sexual orientation conversion therapists and analysis of psychotherapy sessions by independent third party observers. The current paper reports on a segment of data from a larger study of sexual orientation conversion therapy (Shidlo and Schroeder, 2001).

Participants' Perception of the Study

Sexual orientation conversion therapy is a controversial and socially sensitive issue (cf. ABC News, 1998; Miller, 2000). Therefore, participants' perception of the research and researchers both before, during, and after the interview is a critical variable. In our case, the pre-interview perception of participants was affected by the *original* name of the study: "Homophobic Therapies: Documenting the Damage." Our initial goal in this study was to document negative effects and harm of conversion therapies (an area that had not been empirically studied, though it has been identified as a priority topic for research [cf. American Psychiatric Association, 2000; Haldeman, 2001]). After pilot interviews, we discovered that some participants who reported feeling harmed also reported feeling helped. We were contacted by participants who reported positive benefits only. *We then decided to broaden our inquiry by actively recruiting participants who felt helped as well as harmed.* After we changed the project name to a more inclusive one–"Changing Sexual Orientation: Does Counseling Work?"–we were contacted by additional participants who had felt helped by these interventions. (For a report on the subset of participants who felt helped by conversion therapies, see Shidlo and Schroeder, 2001.)

Many participants were curious about our own views on sexual orientation conversion therapies. We told them that we are openly gay psychologists and that our research was hosted by two gay organizations: the National Lesbian and Gay Health Association and the National Gay and Lesbian Task Force. At the end of each interview we asked the respondent about their perception of bias in the structured interview or any information that they may have heard about our investigation. Responses fell into two categories: no prior knowledge about the study or perception of bias; and *pre-interview* perception of a "pro-gay" bias, or concern that we may be affiliated with a religious organization or ex-gay group. Both groups reported that they felt the interview had allowed them to articulate their recollection of conversion therapy.

> [I was] very happy with the interview. I had no idea of your bias and felt you were very fair.

> I was hoping that . . . because I saw this was sponsored by the gay and lesbian center [sic], I was hoping this would truly be an unbiased study.

> Before [the interview], I thought, well, maybe you were looking for something and not wanting to hear what I had to say. But I felt like it's been very unbiased, and you listened. I feel you said that I [the interviewer] want to make sure you got your feelings down right. So I feel real comfortable with it.

When participants asked whether we could assure them of the fairness and lack of bias of our research, we told them that the design, execution or report of results was never influenced by the hosting organizations.

A related methodological issue affecting the quality of data is participants' feeling of safety during the interview. It is critical that they feel comfortable to speak freely about intimate and sometimes painful or embarrassing information about their attempts to change sexual orientation. We believe that this is an especially critical issue in research on conversion therapy, because many of our interviewees reported withholding information or fabricating information when discussing changes in their sexual orientation with their conversion therapists (Shidlo and Schroeder, 2001). With regard to their experience of the interview, our participants reported:

> I think your interview was very good. I didn't feel pressured or threatened to say certain things. It allowed me to be honest.

> It's hard to talk about it now and remember . . . It's embarrassing to talk about it . . .

> I was a little apprehensive and nervous about the interview. . . . It's tough, talking about things like this not easy for me at all, I, I'm trying to be as honest as I can with you, it's very difficult . . . in just trying to think back to thoughts that came to my head, they're difficult, trying to be accurate and honest as I can be. I'm looking for answers myself.

Sample and Procedure

Participants Inclusionary and Exclusionary Criteria

Structured interviews were conducted between 1995 and 2000. For the segment of data reported in this paper, participants who met the following criteria were included: (a) history of at least six sessions in sexual orientation conversion therapy with a licensed clinician; and (b) pre-treatment self-report of 5 to 7 (more homosexual than heterosexual to exclusively homosexual) on a modified 7-point Kinsey scale (Kinsey, Pomeroy, and Martin, 1948) assessing sexual desire, attraction, and feelings. We defined sexual orientation conversion therapy as any intervention administered by a licensed psychologist, psychiatrist, social worker, family and marriage therapist, or counselor which the consumer viewed as being explicitly aimed at changing a homosexual orientation.

Because of social sensitivity to questions about sexuality in general and homosexual orientations in particular, no pre-screening was conducted. Instead, we interviewed all individuals who contacted us reporting a history of any kind of sexual orientation conversion intervention. The total number of interviews conducted was 216. Fifty-two were excluded from the current analysis because these participants reported that they attended para-professional conversion interventions only (see Shidlo and Schroeder, 2001 for a report on these participants). Fourteen additional interviews were excluded from the final analysis because the participant: (a) had less than six sessions of a conversion intervention (4); (b) reported 1 to 4 (exclusively heterosexual to bisexual) on a modified Kinsey scale (Kinsey et al., 1948) assessing sexual desire, attraction, and feelings (4); (c) did not go through an intervention explicitly aimed at changing homosexual orientation (1); (d) immersed himself in self-help conversion material but did not undergo a formal intervention (3); (e) was hard of hearing and had difficulty following structured interview (1); and (f) appeared to have a thought disorder (1).

Sample Characteristics

The number of participants included in this report was 150. Eleven (9%) of participants were female, 139 (93%) were male. Participants' mean age was 40 years, with a SD of 11.6 and range from 20 to 74. With regard to ethnicity, 128 (85%) participants were Caucasian, 8 Latino (5%), 1 (< 1%) African American, and 3 (2%) Asian American. Ninety-seven participants (65%) considered themselves religious and 33 (22%) non-religious; 85 participants identified with a Christian based faith, nine Jewish, two Pagan, and one Buddhist. Percentages do not add up to 100% because of missing data.

Participants reported receiving psychotherapy from a total of 203 practitioners: 122 psychologists (16 of whom were identified by the participant as religiously oriented therapists), 32 psychiatrists, 22 social workers (4 religiously identified), 11 marriage and family counselors (4 religiously identified), and 16 M.A. level therapists (5 religiously identified). Many participants reported courses of therapy with different practitioners.

Procedure

For the first two years of the study, participants were recruited through advertising in gay and lesbian web sites and e-mail lists. Upon receiving funding from the H. van Ameringen foundation in June 1997, we were able to embark on a national advertising campaign for recruiting participants. Neutral advertisements were placed nationally in gay and non-gay press, a web site for the study was established and direct mailings were sent to both gay and ex-gay organizations and to a national professional group of conversion therapists. A toll-free phone number was established to facilitate access by potential participants.

At the start of each 90-minute interview, participants were given an informed consent form; when the interview was conducted by telephone, verbal consent was obtained. If the interview was tape-recorded, additional consent was obtained. At the end of the interview, participants were offered the opportunity to see results of the study and to give feedback on the interview itself.

Four doctoral level psychologists were utilized for the administration of the structured interview. Interviewers were trained and supervised by the researchers. Most of the interviews were conducted by Schroeder and Shidlo. The researchers randomly reviewed audio tapes to confirm that the protocol was being observed.

Measures

A semi-structured protocol was used. Since this was an exploratory study with an emphasis on qualitative data, the protocol evolved through several iterations during the course of our study (for a discussion of the rationale of using iteration in research, see Rubin and Rubin, 1995). As interviews were completed, we identified new critical areas of questioning which were integrated into subsequent interviews.

The protocol included the following areas of inquiry:

- *Goals of treatment.* What were the goals and were they mutually agreed upon with the therapist? Was there a specific request to have sexual orientation changed?
- *Information about homosexuality and treatment.* What information was provided by the clinician about gay people and the gay communities? How was homosexuality framed by the counselor (e.g., mental disorder, developmental disorder, addiction, sin or spiritual disorder, learned behavior, sexual brokenness, caused by abuse, normal sexuality)? This was followed by a question on how the therapist explained the participant's homosexual orientation. Other questions included how the counselor explained the counseling would help the participant.
- *Emotional responses to information.* How did the participant feel when the framework for understanding the cause of his homosexual orientation was explained?
- *Informed consent.* Did the clinician provide information about possible therapy consequences, both positive and negative, of the intervention, explore the two APAs' positions on homosexuality, and explore treatment options including gay-affirmative treatment?
- *Intervention type.* What occurred in the treatment sessions and what was the approach to change?

• *Help versus harm.* Participants were asked open- and close-ended questions about perceived help and harm of each intervention they reported.

RESULTS AND DISCUSSION

The structure of this section is as follows: (a) representation of the APAs' positions on the scientific understanding of a homosexual orientation; (b) informed consent; (c) confidentiality; (d) the relationship between religion and conversion therapy; and (e) appropriate termination.

How the Two APAs Decisions Were Represented

We asked respondents whether their therapists told them that the American Psychological Association and the American Psychiatric Association do not view a homosexual orientation as a psychological disorder or mental illness. We distinguished between psychotherapies conducted before and after the year of declassification of homosexuality (1973) by the American Psychiatric Association. On this variable, we have information on 120 participants who reported on 149 *post-1973* conversion therapy courses (some individuals went through more than one conversion therapy). Participants reported only 38 instances (26%) where clinicians informed them of the APAs' positions. In these instances two salient themes emerged: (a) the APAs' views were based on political pressure from the gay community; and (b) the APAs' views were not based on empirical research. For example, one participant said: "[my therapist] felt like it was political pressure that had caused the APA to change it, rather than research. That there were militant pro-gay people who forced the change." Similarly, another participant reports that his therapist told him that "The APA was pressured politically into changing the diagnosis, but actually it still is a disorder. But the only reason they changed it was because they were politically pressured by protests of gay groups and such." One participant reported that his therapist told him the American Psychiatric Association's decision to de-pathologize homosexuality was "a tragedy." Another respondent said that he spoke to his therapist about his reading "a lot of stuff that says being gay is fine that there is no mental illness. He [the therapist] was very dismissive of it. He said it was more of like a political activism of the gay movement as opposed to any psychological model."

Other therapists seemed to view the APAs' decisions on homosexuality as secular information that should not have bearing on religion-based psychotherapy. These therapists told participants that religious values supersede secular and scientific attitudes and knowledge. One participant recalls that his therapist mentioned the APAs' decisions on homosexuality "in the context of why it was important for me to see a Christian psychologist, because all psychologists are not Christian."

In conclusion, according to client reports, some conversion therapists may not be informing patients that the APAs do not view a homosexual orientation as a psychological disorder. Others who discuss this with patients may be misrepresenting the scientific basis for the APAs' views on a homosexual orientation.

Informed Consent

Informed consent is an integral part of the ethical practice of psychotherapy (O'Neill, 1998). Standard 4.02 (APA, 1992, p. 1605), titled "Informed Consent to Therapy," instructs psychologists to provide patients with significant information concerning the proposed intervention. Clarification is provided by the American Psychological Association document, "Guidelines for Psychotherapy" (2000), where psychologists are reminded that "Based on the APA Ethics Code, the 'Appropriate Therapeutic Responses to Sexual Orientation' policy calls on psychologists to discuss the treatment, its theoretical basis, reasonable outcomes, and alternative treatment approaches" (p. 1443). Our data strongly suggest that, in the area of informed consent, many conversion therapists may not be practicing in a manner consistent with the APA Ethics Code (1992).

In the subsequent section we identify several areas of informed consent relevant to conversion therapy followed by illustrative examples from our interviews with consumers. The areas of informed consent we examine are:

- Did the clinician provide accurate information about sexual orientation?
- Did the clinician provide accurate information about the proposed intervention and prognosis?
- Were other treatment options discussed?
- Was there coercion in the therapy?

Did the Clinician Provide Accurate Information About Sexual Orientation?

The APA Ethics Code instructs "psychologists . . . [not to] make false or deceptive statements concerning . . . the scientific or clinical basis for . . . their services" (APA, 1992, Standard 3.03(a), p. 1604). The most frequent violation of informed consent guidelines, based on our sample of conversion therapy consumers' reports, was a failure to provide accurate and scientific information about homosexuality. Participants were told by their therapists or counselors that: (a) homosexuality is in itself a psychological disorder or is a symptom of another disorder; (b) homosexuality does not exist; and that (c) gay lives are inherently unhappy. Defaming and fraudulent information about lesbians and gay men is contradicted by widely available psychological research (cf. Anderson and Adley, 1997; D'Augelli and Patterson, 1995; Gonsiorek, 1991; Perez, Debord, and Bieschke, 2000). The propagation of inaccurate information on lesbians and gay men by conversion therapists represents a failure to uphold standard 1.05 of the APA Ethics Code (1992) which calls on psychologists to "maintain a reasonable level of awareness of current scientific and professional information in their fields of activity, and undertake ongoing efforts to maintain competence in the skills they use" (p. 1600). The following are examples of some of the misinformation provided by conversion therapists:

Claims That Homosexuality Is a Psychological Disorder
in Itself or a Symptom of Another Disorder

Many participants reported that their therapist told them that their homosexual orientation was a psychological or developmental disorder. One participant stated, "for those guys [conversion therapists], it's always your mother's fault. He wouldn't say it exactly like that, but we always talked about mother issues. . . . [that it was a] developmental issue, that I had learned to love a woman, but not to love her sexually, because you're not supposed to love your mom sexually." Another participant said that his therapist told him that his homosexuality "was the result of my domineering mother and absent father and that I was searching for a connection to the masculine and that it had been fused incorrectly with sexuality. I needed to connect with men in a non-sexual manner as this was the route to healing." A clinician told a respondent that homosexuality was a disease that could be cured through aversion therapy:

> [He said] if you didn't do this you would go insane or kill yourself. . . . He called it a short circuit . . . what the chemicals in the body do, does not necessarily condone what you should be aroused to. But they are shorting out and making me aroused to men and not women. . . . therapy would help me get over that endorphin, it would train my body to relate to the scent of a woman as erotic, as opposed to a scent of men. That kind of scientific mumbo jumbo.

Other conversion therapists told patients that their homosexuality is a symptom of a psychiatric disorder. A participant reported that his therapist diagnosed him as suffering from obsessive-compulsive disorder and sexual addiction because of his homosexuality. He said, "I was not allowed to be gay-defined so . . . [the therapist] termed it sexual addiction even though I had never had sex." Another participant reported:

> My therapist believes that a large part of homosexuality is caused by not being able to process or access authentic emotion. By doing so, and by

learning how to do so, that in fulfilling a lot of the emotional needs left over from whenever, positively, that homosexuality can diminish.

Interestingly, some participants recounted that their therapists would insist on a putative etiology for their homosexuality even when the patient denied the existence of any such events in their history. For example, several participants reported that their therapist identified the cause of their homosexuality as a supposed history of child abuse, even in the absence of memories or evidence for such abuse:

> He was making assumptions that I was molested as a child. I was never molested by anyone. *He said I must have been molested.*

> There was also an attempt to explain this as being sexual abuse although I was never abused and he tried to convince me that I was sexually abused when I was a small baby. He made these conclusions from drawings I had made.

> I had already assumed the cause to be my mother and father. When he tried to convince me I was abused and this was the cause I became angry and terminated the treatment.

> I was discouraged. The therapy was not being effective and the therapist was trying to fabricate a history of sexual abuse when it did not exist.

One participant spoke of feeling that his therapist was overly influenced by a pre-existing model of homosexuality and as a result was not hearing him accurately: "The last half of the private sessions I began saying things he expected to hear. The questions he would ask, *he never seemed to listen that I wasn't fitting in a pattern he expected.*"

Other participants felt that their therapist would magnify the importance of events in their lives to explain their homosexuality. One participant reported that he had a good relationship with his father. Nonetheless, his therapist said that conversion therapy "would help me deal with any injustice that I felt my father showed me. [He said] I could work through that problem and heal the wounds and be okay. *I didn't think there were any big wounds to heal.*"

Homosexuality Does Not Exist

Some participants reported that they were told by their therapists that their homosexual orientation did not exist. On this variable, we have information from 73 participants who reported on 94 courses of conversion therapy. Fifty-nine clinicians (63%) were reported to have told participants that they are not *really* homosexual. Clients were frequently told that they had always been heterosexual in some form and just needed to re-discover their true (hetero) sexuality.

> [He said there was] no such thing as a true homosexual. People were just confused and had a mental disorder that had to be cured.

> The therapist said that homosexuality did not exist. Only in a perverse form in people who did not like themselves.

> The therapist said that I was absolutely heterosexual.

> The psychologist said that I struggled with homosexuality and that I didn't want to be gay. He said: you're not gay; you're homophobic. He said I feared it so much that I was afraid I was. It made me question my feelings. I have an attraction for men, none for women, I told him that. Made me question what does it mean to be gay? I was really confused. I didn't understand how I could not be gay. He said he didn't think there was anything to change, that I just thought I was gay. That I wasn't really, he said I wasn't gay.

> My therapists kept telling me I was straight yet I knew that I was gay. Things did not match. The mixed messages from the therapists were the most damaging of all. I still am coping with this.

> He followed the standard LDS [The Church of Jesus Christ of *Latter-Day Saints*] line which was that homosexuality did not exist and there was no such thing as a homosexual. God made you heterosexual. God does not create homosexuals therefore homosexuality does not exist.

These findings are consistent with the research of Nystrom (1997) who found that one-third of gay men and lesbians surveyed said their therapist "refused to acknowledge" their sexual orientation or dismissed it as a phase that would eventually pass.

Gay Lives Are Inherently Unhappy

Almost all of our participants were told by their therapists that gay persons' lives and relationships are undesirable, unhealthy, and unhappy. A clinician prominent for his work in conversion therapy told a patient at their final telephone therapy session: "Remember you'll never be happy gay and never find fulfillment in another man." Earlier in treatment this same clinician said: "Why would you like to stick your penis in something that represents death like an anus, where shit comes out, versus where you can have it where life is, a vagina." Another respondent reports that when he told his therapist that he had read about "gay couples who are happy," the therapist responded, "I have never known a single gay person to be happy." Similar prejudiced and unscientifically based comments were made by other therapists:

> [The therapist said] homosexuality is a compulsive behavior, maybe not in the beginning, but 10 years down the road it will become compulsive. [He said that] his patients have dreams of 30 cocks in his [sic] face. [He treats] a guy who can't make it to his office without getting sucked five times. . . . [he said that] I had a confused core identity.

> He told me that homosexuals are quite promiscuous, and their lifestyle leads often to drugs, crime, and molestation of children. The usual stereotypes that you hear all the time. He asked me if I had molested my children or had been molested.

> [The] main sell . . . was that it inevitably lead you to an unhappy lonely life . . . He knew of no gay couples that lasted for significant time, and he knew no gay people who were happy or adjusted. He was also implying that there was something weak or mentally unhealthy too, by the way he described it, the way he was asking me about my sexual history, and the way he talked about how it could be changed. It sort of implied a mental illness model.

> [The therapist said] that gay people all get AIDS and that I can avoid hardship through leading a heterosexual lifestyle.

> He [the therapist] wanted me to read books . . . describing the gay lifestyle, how lonely and depressing [it was], no hope, *he wanted me to internalize that and make sure I knew that it was absolutely the worst, and I need to always think that* . . . He knew the one thing that pushed a lot of buttons. . . . [that I] wanted to . . . have a monogamous relationship. Settle down with woman for rest of our lives. He was showing and pushing that guys in the gay community are all very promiscuous, they have millions of partners, you will never get what you are looking for, monogamy with one guy. You will always be on the search and prowl. You would always be disappointed and depressed that these guys would leave you for another guy. That there was no stability, no true love.

Conclusion

Many conversion therapists appear to be providing patients false and prejudicial information on gay men and lesbians. In fact, there appears to be a significant element of propagandizing by some conversion therapists on the supposed horrors of life as a gay man or lesbian. Our data from participants who were in conversion therapy are consistent with the American Psychiatric Association (1998) finding that "Many patients who have undergone 'reparative therapy' relate that they were inaccurately told that homosexuals are lonely, unhappy individuals who never achieve acceptance or satisfaction." Garnets and her colleagues (1991) and Nystrom (1997) have similarly documented many incidents of anti-gay bias among therapists. These findings are consistent with descriptions of gay men and lesbians' lives in the conversion therapy literature itself (Nicolosi, 1993; Satinover, 1996; Siegel, 1988; Socarides, 1978, 1995; van den Aardweg, 1997). For example, Nicolosi (1993), a founder of the National Association for Research and Therapy of Homosexuality (NARTH), writes: "Homosexual relationships are so characteristically volatile because the homosexual hates what he loves" (p. 152). Stern (Nicolosi, 1999a) views lesbians and gay men as "not having grown up"; he says: "The homosexual often fears otherness, and in this fear, may beckon to an idealized image of himself–'Be me, and I'll be you.' The world becomes an eternal playground, and growth is stymied." Satinover (Nicolosi, 1999b), who testified before Congress against legalizing gay marriage, has said: "Homosexuality . . . is a method of adapting to adverse circumstances. But like sociopathy, it exacts a cost in terms of constrictions of relationships. . . . I believe homosexuality–like narcissism–is best viewed as a spiritual and moral illness."

Patients in conversion therapy may not be advised about scientific or psychological information on gay, lesbian and bisexual individuals, relationships, and communities. Instead, they may be exposed to prejudice and falsehoods. This violates Standard 1.06 of the APA Ethics Code (1992) which states that "Psychologists rely on scientifically and professionally derived knowledge when making scientific or professional judgments or when engaging in scholarly or professional endeavors."

Did the Clinician Provide Accurate Information About the Proposed Intervention and Prognosis?

In this provision of informed consent, clinicians discuss with patients how they think a proposed intervention will be helpful. Informed consent for conversion therapy should include information about the workings and efficacy of the procedure. In addition to linking the procedure to the putative causes of a homosexual orientation, the clinician should offer a prognosis, and list any possible side-effects.

A question about whether consumers were informed about the possible negative effects of conversion therapy was introduced late in our study. Therefore, we have data from only 22 participants who reported on 47 courses of conversion therapies. Participants reported that only four clinicians (9%) informed them of possible negative effects of the intervention. Our findings also suggest that some therapists misled clients with:

- Unfounded prognoses based on patient personality characteristics.
- Assurances that a shift in sexual orientation is likely if clients are highly motivated and work hard in the treatment.
- Misrepresentations of the scientific evidence supporting the efficacy of the proposed intervention.

Unfounded Prognoses Based on Patient Personality Characteristics

Many of our participants reported that their therapists had informed them that they were promising candidates for change. They were told that prototype for a successful candidate for conversion therapy was an individual who possessed stereotypical male (for men) or female (for women) personality features, had little or no same-sex sexual history, had strong religious faith, did not identify as gay or lesbian, did not have gay friends, and who asserted a strong motivation to change. We have found no empirical data that demonstrates that these characteristics support a good prognosis for changing homosexual orientation.

> My parents basically got a promise from him that he would change me to straight. [He told my parents] that he had a lot of success and he could [help me] *if I was straight-acting enough.* . . . He would first have to interview me and see. He gave them a promise. Then I went in and had my first session. He listened to my story. He said *I was probably one of the best candidates for change. Not only that I had a strong religious belief system, and strong family support, and much more masculine and straight attributes than gay people. And that I hadn't accepted any of the identity of being gay.* He said I had a lot of hope and he said he didn't think it would be a problem for me to become straight. I asked him how long? He said about a year . . . that since I didn't latch on to the term gay and didn't identify with being gay, I was definitely a straight person, that something had developmentally . . . in my life gone wrong, and I could overcome it, it would be all fine and dandy at the end.

> He [the therapist] said "all of your tests and experiences show that I have good news for you. They indicate that you are straight, that you are not

gay and that we have a few things to work through and everything will be fine." I'd wake up 17 years later and realize I am still gay.

Assurance That a Shift in Sexual Orientation Is Likely If Clients Are Highly Motivated and Work Hard in the Treatment

Many respondents reported that their therapists assured them of the success of conversion therapy if they were motivated and compliant with the intervention. These findings are consistent with NARTH's claim that, although change in sexual orientation usually takes "several years," the "keys to change are *desire, persistence,* and a willingness to investigate the *conscious* and *unconscious conflicts* from which the condition originated" (NARTH, undated document B, italics in the original). There is no empirical evidence to support the claim that the outcome of conversion therapy is associated with the level of the patient's motivation. In fact, our own work (Shidlo and Schroeder, 2001) documents that many individuals with exceedingly high levels of motivation and compliance with conversion therapies, in treatment for periods of over 10 years, failed to change their sexual orientation. The following are typical examples of respondents who were told that their motivation and compliance were the keys to success in conversion therapy:

> If I worked hard enough and trusted God enough, I would have these pathways in the brain, these habits, would be healed over, corrected or removed. And if I stuck with it long enough, it would automatically occur. Kind of like, being straight is the normal way, if you work hard enough and realize these pathways were causing it, eventually you would come back to place where you would be back to normal.

> He was more optimistic, he said the sky is the limit. *I could change as much as I was willing to work.*

> If my needs for male bonding were met my attractions would go away. *He said, anybody can escape homosexuality if you work hard enough.*

> [He said] that *it could be overcome, that I just needed to want to [change] bad enough, that I had to trust in God, and believe that God didn't create me this way,* that I was created in his image. [It was] a big play on my religious beliefs.

The psychological consequence of being told that hard work was a sufficient condition for changing sexual orientation is that clients who failed attributed the failure to themselves and came to believe that they were ineffectual and lazy. One respondent says: "It seemed to not be working and he would always tell me that I was not trying hard enough . . . that was the worst part."

*Misrepresentation of the Scientific Evidence Supporting
the Efficacy of the Proposed Intervention*

A wide array of psychotherapies and behavioral procedures were presented by therapists to our participants as efficacious in changing a homosexual orientation. Interventions were presented together with a putative theory of the causes of a homosexual orientation. Proposed treatments included combinations of: (a) cognitive behavior therapy, (b) behavior therapy, (c) psychoanalysis, (d) aversive conditioning, and (e) covert sensitization. Many of these interventions also included a religious component. However, conversion therapists who tell their patients that these interventions are efficacious in changing their sexual orientation are disregarding the scientific consensus about the empirical data (APA, 1998, 2000; American Psychiatric Association, 1998, 2000; Davison, 1991; Drescher, 2001a; Gonsiorek, 1991; Haldeman, 1991, 1994; Martin, 1984).

We asked participants: "Did your counselor(s) tell you that s/he could make you become heterosexual or bisexual?" One hundred sixty-seven participants gave us information in this area on 167 clinicians. Of these, 112 (67%) therapists told them that therapy would help them become heterosexual or bisexual.

Toward the end of the study, we introduced a question asking whether clients were informed about the possibility that the intervention may not be successful in changing sexual orientation. A small data set is available for this variable from 23 participants who reported on 47 therapy courses. Participants reported that 18 (38%) therapists told them of the possibility that the intervention may not be successful in changing sexual orientation.

Our participants reported that they were offered the following interventions to change their sexual orientation:

Cognitive-Behavior and Behavior Therapy. Procedures included thought-stopping, aversion therapy (electric shock and noxious chemical), covert sensitization, systematic desensitization, modeling, shaping, and operant-conditioning. The following illustrate what participants were told by their therapists about these interventions:

> He felt it was a behavioral thing. . . . Like a Pavlov thing. By aversion or staying away from it and doing other things it would reinforce the good feelings of the heterosexual feelings and then, by negative things happening to you it would avert the homosexual feelings.

> He told me that in his experience he found that once he was able to get the patient to become comfortable with females, the homosexual issues went away.

Being around other men will help me get the validation from men that I need from non-sexual relationships and then I would pursue relationships with women.

If I made friends with heterosexual men, I would find myself attracted to women. It would help you lessen the homosexual attraction and put you in relationship with men and women so that . . . you become one of the boys, you would find yourself being attracted to the opposite-sex. To heal the masculine wound or hurt inflicted by men on you.

That . . . [the therapy] would show me how the emotional deficits occurred and how I could learn how to fill those correctly. By taking appropriate action through proper socialization and proper heterosexual activities I could therefore become heterosexual.

The therapist . . . didn't think I was gay and made that comment to me, I guess it was part of behavior modification. He said if you want to be like a man act like a man, start buying girly magazines and that will take your mind off men.

In aversion shock therapy the idea was to train us to respond erotically to women and fear an erotic response to males.

Aversive treatment where I was brought into a room and exposed to sexually explicit stimuli of pictures of naked men and injected with some substance which would induce vomiting [This participant reported that he got no support or guidance from the clinician].

Some participants were instructed in procedures to make them more stereotypically masculine or feminine. Men were encouraged to engage in team-sports, to go the gym, and to attend Promise Keepers[5] workshops. Women were encouraged to learn how to cook, sew, and apply make-up. One respondent was told by his therapist to stop playing the piano and change his course of music studies because "playing the piano is what makes you gay." The participant was told that if he discontinued playing the piano his homosexual attraction would be extinguished. Another male participant was encouraged to get married: "[the therapist said] that I could be happy with a woman. That's what I needed to do was to distract myself from the homosexuality, that I needed to get married. That I would be so focused on the family that the homosexuality could atrophy and go away."

Additional cognitive and behavioral interventions employed included tying one's hand to the bedpost to avoid masturbating, using sexual surrogates, imagining getting AIDS when aroused by the same-sex, masturbating to gay pornography to minimize having actual sex with same-gender partners, abstaining from masturbation, using the HALT technique (framing same sex desire as being the result of feeling *H*ungry, *A*ngry, *L*onely or *T*ired), employing EMDR and hypnosis.

Psychodynamic Therapy. Participants who underwent psychodynamic therapies were told by their therapist that homosexuality is caused by faulty family dynamics. Therapists implied that if a patient understood the etiology of their homosexuality, they could make the necessary behavioral adjustments that would lead to its cessation. For example, one participant stated that his therapist told him his homosexual orientation "was a result of my domineering mother and absent father and that I was searching for a connection to the masculine which had been fused incorrectly with sexuality. I needed to connect with men in a non-sexual manner as this was the route to healing." Another participant explained, "it was a whole system of unmet needs, through exploring relationships I had with my father and men in general. . . . basically I never had real good relationships with men, or was always intimidated by men, the type of men I was attracted to was to a body image I wanted to achieve myself. If I found healthy ways to meet these needs, the homosexuality would go away or lessen over time."

Psychotropic Intervention. Psychotropic medications were employed either on their own or combined with conversion psychotherapy. Patients were prescribed anti-depressants and anxiolytics to help them control their homosexual behavior or to reduce their sexual fantasy life and desire:

> I would be medicated and dull my sexual desire. He said it would take two to three years. [I received] psychotherapy combined with medications to control my fantasies and control my masturbation. I was to follow a 12-step program for sexual addicts in a workbook. I had never had sex with another man up until that point, yet he diagnosed me as a sex addict.

> This would take a lot of hard work and commitment to not be gay. . . . Medication would help . . . nothing much more specific than that.

> I was gay. I was given all sorts of hormonal therapies to make me into a straight guy.

> He gave me Valium to treat my anxiety about my sexual orientation.

Religion-Based Psychotherapy. Many of the religion-based therapies incorporated numerous adaptations of interventions such as cognitive-behavioral therapy and behavior therapy. Testimonials, mentoring, prayer, Bible readings, and Christian weekend workshops were reported by our participants.

Some therapists introduced religious beliefs into the conversion therapy. One participant reports, "He thought if I dealt with my abuse issues and my misconception about God and the Bible . . . I had come from a fundamental background, that was the reason I thought I was gay, because of a guilt complex about God. If I investigated that stuff, I would realize I wasn't gay." Another respondent said, "His view was that once you understood your childhood and the pain of the relationship with your parents and let God in you could be changed by this and you then become attracted to women. If you could learn to do something masculine you could then eventually internalize this and become straight."

Were Other Treatment Options Discussed?

Although not explicitly mandated by the APA Ethics Code (1992), there is a growing recognition that discussing alternative treatments is an inherent part of true consent (APA, 2001; O'Neill, 1998). We asked participants: "Did your counselor(s) tell you that there are licensed mental health practitioners who do not treat homosexuality as a disorder, but rather help people feel less shame and distress about it?" Information for this variable is available on 118 participants who reported on 164 conversion therapy courses conducted as of 1974. Participants reported that only 27 clinicians (17%) advised them of the availability of therapists who are not biased against a homosexual orientation.

A second question asked was: "Did your counselor(s) encourage and support you to explore the option of going to a gay-affirmative practitioner who wouldn't try to change your orientation?" Information on this variable is available for 118 participants who reported on 166 courses of conversion therapies. Only four clinicians discussed with their clients the option of seeking therapy from a practitioner who would not try to change sexual orientation.

> By not giving me accurate information and telling me there were other options and choices he did a big disservice as a professional with the power of his role as psychologist and professor. Telling me it was the right thing to do took me on journey that lasted longer than it should have . . . it created more pain for me and my wife than it had to. I trusted him [when] he said it would work.

> It was not a choice. Either you will be gay and unhappy or stick with me and change.

> It made . . . me angry that he wouldn't give me a choice. . . . it was his way or the highway. It just hurt because I felt down deep that I needed to have the option of accepting myself as a gay man. When I saw him, I didn't

have that option. If I wanted to keep seeing him I had to go straight. I had no option.

I said I'd really want to continue the marriage, and I said, wasn't there something I could do, take drugs or something? He said the only way to change the feelings was this electroshock therapy.

I flat-out refused to do the shock therapy. He said he couldn't do anything for me because I wouldn't cooperate.

The therapist . . . didn't suggest that I would want to stay that way [i.e., gay]; it was never an option [to] . . . learn to accept it.

Was There Coercion in the Therapy?

The issue of coercion came up in two ways: Coercion by therapists and coercion by religious universities.

Coercion by therapists. Several participants spoke of pressure by their therapist to go to the media to tell of their success in changing sexual orientation. For example, one participant said: "We were encouraged a lot to tell the media about our alleged change. We were encouraged to go on Jerry Springer . . . he [the therapist] was a media-hound." Another participant, who ultimately failed conversion therapy, reported that his clinician, a nationally known conversion therapist, encouraged him to take part in a panel in an ex-gay conference to present his successful struggle with homosexuality. When we asked what it was like to be asked to appear with his therapist on a panel, the participant said: "I was very honored. I wanted to be poster child for NARTH. I believed in the cause so strongly." The same participant reports that his therapist referred him to our research project on conversion therapy, but was told not to reveal that he had been referred by this NARTH clinician. "He wanted people who would give a good report . . . [He said] call this number and say a friend sent you, don't say NARTH sent you."

Coercion by religious universities. Some of our participants were forced by religious universities to pursue conversion therapy subsequent to: (a) the student confiding in their advisor, (b) being identified by another student as gay, (c) being caught having sex on university premises, or (d) being entrapped by campus security. The penalty for not complying with the order to attend conversion therapy was expulsion from the university.

What are the ethical issues facing practitioners employed by an academic institution that requires conversion therapy for lesbian and gay students at the threat of academic expulsion? Should they provide conversion therapy for students who are mandated to attend? Do psychologists who engage in such practices violate the 1975 American Psychological Association statement (Conger, 1975, p. 633) opposing discrimination against lesbians and gay men? Does providing conversion therapy under coercive circumstances, violate section 4.02 on informed consent of the APA Ethics Code (1992) which states that patients express consent freely and without undue influence?

For example, one participant we interviewed was a student at a large religious university. He says, "I am being forced to be in therapy. I sit there and agree with what he has to say to avoid confrontation. He is pushing me to marry a woman. My goal is basically just to graduate." Another student was entrapped at his school: "I responded to a note on a bathroom wall, and was caught by campus security. They sent me to one of the counselors. . . . This therapy is currently being mandated by . . . [large religious university] as a condition for me to continue and graduate . . . This therapist is a Nazi and is more radical about it. It focuses on early childhood and on my relationship with my father."

Conclusion

Many conversion therapists may be treating patients without obtaining full informed consent. This study found serious causes for concern in the areas of providing misinformation about sexual orientation, misrepresenting the efficacy of conversion therapies and their prognoses, and failure to discuss treatment options.

These issues are raised in the light of our findings that many participants in conversion therapies who fail to change sexual orientation appear to suffer significant psychological harm (Shidlo and Schroeder, 2001). It is troubling that many conversion therapists do not appear to discuss with their patients the possibility that there may be side-effects or harm from these procedures. These findings are consistent with a review of the conversion therapy literature, which, on the whole, neglects the issue of harm completely (for a further examination of this point see Drescher, 2001a, b; Haldeman, 2001).

NARTH, an organization representing conversion therapists, has said that conversion therapy should be provided only to those who seek it freely: "We believe that treatment should be offered to those who voluntarily seek it" and "acknowledge that many homosexual men and women do not wish to change their psychosexual adaption, and we respect their wishes not to seek therapy. . . ." (NARTH, undated document A). However, some therapists are providing conversion therapy under coercive situations–for example, lesbian and gay students are being forced into treatment or face expulsion from their religious academic institutions.

Confidentiality

Violations of confidentiality were reported primarily among participants who received treatment within a religious university or an affiliated counseling setting. Such violations included divulging information to school officials and speaking with the (adult) patient's parents without consent. According to the APA Ethics Code (1992, p. 1606) Standard 4.09, "psychologists have a primary obligation and take reasonable precautions to respect the confidentiality rights of those with whom they work or consult, recognizing that confidentiality may be established by law, institutional rules, or professional or scientific relationships." Moreover, "psychologists disclose confidential information without the consent of the individual only as mandated by law, or where permitted by law for a valid purpose . . . "

Several participants reported a breach of confidentiality between their therapist and school officials. Some suffered academic consequences as a result of a school official being told by the university clinician about the content of the conversion therapy: "I ended up being thrown out from school because the counselor, who was married to the Dean of students, told him [the Dean] about the [sexual] incident that happened between me and my roommate in the dormitory. They wanted me to be healed and have God's forgiveness. . . . they kicked me out of school." Another respondent reports that when he went to a school therapist at a Christian college he was told: "You know that homosexual behavior is against the rules of the school. If you do anything and I know about it, I will tell them and they will kick you out." This resulted in the student both fearing therapy and feeling that his sexual orientation was demeaned: "I stopped seeing him. He wanted me to come back, but I didn't trust him. I felt like, this is how I'm viewed, how the lifestyle is viewed by the school. I didn't seem to know what to do with it."

Failure to maintain confidentiality was also reported by consumers of therapy in private practice settings. An adult participant reported that, to his surprise, his father arrived one day at his session: "My dad came in invited not by me but by the therapist, and apologized for not being a good father . . . Saying I wasn't gay because I had an overbearing mother . . . " Another patient states that the clinician "proceeded to tell my dad about my sexual history. This was after assuring me of confidentiality . . . including mentioning names [of men the participant had had sex with]." A married man who had been in conversion treatment reports that the clinician would give unsolicited updates on the treatment to the participant's wife without his consent, "He would talk to my wife, he had sessions with her once a month, updates, on the progress with me." And another participant states that, "Although it was supposed to be confidential, the counselor's son was my age. We went on a retreat together. He [the counselor] told his son. Things hit the wall. Even my parents were upset. We agreed that nothing was changing or getting fixed."

Conclusion

Clinicians employed at religious universities that expel lesbian and gay students, when told by patients about their homosexual orientation, may have a conflict of interest. Some of them may be in ethical violation of patient confidentiality. General knowledge of this may discourage lesbian and gay students from seeking psychotherapy at university settings. Conversion therapists in private settings may involve family members in the treatment of their lesbian and gay patient without sufficient consideration of the clinical and ethical issues involved. Clinicians who treat patients whose therapy is paid for by the church may need to consider carefully the *clinical* consequences of sharing information with church officials, *even when consent is obtained*. For example, one respondent, who consented that his therapist share treatment information with his Bishop, reports that he was *consequently not truthful about changes in his sexual orientation with his therapist*. He says:

> [The therapist] told me that because church was paying for it that he would be in contact with my bishop about my progress. That seemed normal. . . . I just wanted the feeling to go away. I wanted to be normal. I loved my wife and wanted these feelings to go away so that I can be a better husband. *I was frantic about not losing my church membership and afraid it would be public and I would be shamed.* I thought if I had to die I would suicide. . . . He offered me shock therapy; I told him I didn't think I was that bad, because the talking helped the feelings go away and I was doing better with my wife. . . . *I went back in the closet and was better about hiding. I convinced the Bishop that I didn't need to go to counseling.* . . . When I look back, I would have quiet and sad times, mourn that it hadn't not worked out. It was so confusing to me.

Religion in Sexual Orientation Conversion Therapy

Psychotherapists are increasingly attending to the importance of a competent integration of religious issues into their clinical work (Bergin, 1991; Richards and Bergin, 2000; Yarhouse and VanOrman, 1999). Supporters of conversion therapy have argued that it is unethical to ignore the central role of religion for some patients who struggle with their homosexual orientation (Throckmorton, 1998; Yarhouse, 1998; Yarhouse and Burkett, 2000). They have written that lack of attention to a patient's religious beliefs is not consistent with the APA Ethics Code (1992) call on psychologists to respect the diversity of patients, including their religion.

The use or introduction of religious beliefs by the therapist into psychotherapy raises challenging questions. Restricting the discussion here to sexual orientation conversion therapies, one hypothesis is that clinicians who introduce religious beliefs into their practice of psychotherapy will have a greater impact, negative or positive, on religious clients. We found in our research that while some participants viewed having a religious clinician as essential in their struggle with their homosexual orientation, others felt adversely impacted. For example one respondent said that his therapist "put the combined imprimatur of the church on homophobia because he had a PhD in psychology." Another clinician who worked for the LDS church told his patient that homosexuality was "a sin, that Satan has taken over you . . . you'll go to hell. Satan wants you to think that you can't change but you can. It's an illness. You need to be cured." Another respondent says: "He [the therapist] of course mixed a lot of religion into it; [he said] we would burn in eternal hell, and the Lord had sent me to him because it was his call in life to help the returning missionaries and members of church who had fallen astray."

Conclusion

Study is needed of the clinical and ethical implications of introducing religion into conversion therapy.

Termination of Conversion Therapy

Not only did many of our participants report a pressure to remain in conversion therapy, they also reported numerous accounts of less than optimal terminations characterized by poor preparation and inadequate treatment referrals. Section 4.09(b) of the APA Ethics Code (1992, p. 1606) states that "(b) Psychologists terminate a professional relationship when it becomes reasonably clear that the patient or client no longer needs the service, is not benefitting, or is being harmed by continued service. (c) Prior to termination for whatever reason, except where precluded by the patient's or client's conduct, the psychologist discusses the patient's or client's views and needs, provides appropriate pre-termination counseling, suggests alternative service providers as appropriate, and takes other reasonable steps to facilitate transfer of responsibility to another provider if the patient or client needs one immediately." In this section, two areas are examined: (a) coercion to remain in conversion therapy; and (b) failure to prepare for termination.

Coercion to Remain in Conversion Therapy

We found several instances of pressure to stay in therapy when a client wanted to leave or was not benefitting from treatment. One participant recounts: "I got accepted to . . . law school. I had to leave and move. Last session I told him that. He thought it was a mistake and that I shouldn't leave therapy. He felt if I left therapy I would not be able to resolve my sexual orientation issues. That was something he didn't want me to do as a mental health professional and as a Christian brother because I would loose my salvation." Another respondent tells of a therapist who pursued contact with him after termination: "I tried to leave him, he wouldn't let me leave. He would call me." A wish to leave because of a lack of progress in therapy was frequently attributed, by the therapist, as a fault of the client for not working hard enough. One conversion therapist told a client that "I hadn't given it enough time. He had seen a lot of progress in me. To leave now would ruin everything, and destroy what I had improved on."

Failure to Prepare for Termination

For most of the participants who terminated conversion therapy as treatment failures, there was a lack of preparation for post-conversion life. Pre-termination counseling neglected: (a) re-entry into gay life; (b) loss of community; and (c) integration of homosexual desire with identity, relationships, and sex. Addressing these issues may be most critical for persons who end conversion therapy as self-perceived failures. This population appears to be more vulnerable to depression, anxiety and self-defeating behaviors (Shidlo and Schroeder, 2001). One participant says of the aftermath of failed conversion therapy: "Instead of getting closer to people I continued to keep it a secret. I felt like I didn't fit in or belong in the gay or straight community. Like I didn't fit anywhere like I was somehow in between. I felt I was afraid to be around gay people, like they would think less of me, because I was naive with no experience whatsoever. . . . in the straight community I had to keep it a secret."

As argued above, conversion therapies include inculcating lesbians and gay men with the belief that a homosexual orientation is a psychological disorder not compatible with a satisfying life. Individuals whose conversion therapies have failed are subsequently left with exaggeratedly negative attitudes toward their own homosexual orientation and without any appropriate tools to cope with either feeling like a failure or how to affirmatively integrate their homosexual orientation into their lives:

> When you have years and years of people telling you it's sick and wrong it wears on you and you start to believe it. I still don't have self-esteem because of negative stuff I've been told my whole life. . . . Because who I am is wrong. If I look in the mirror and I'm not gay or totally straight, where do I fit in? How do I come to terms with that? *They [conversion therapists] never taught me how to deal with that; just how to try and change it.*

Among supporters of conversion therapy, only Yarhouse (1998) has articulated the importance to informed consent of a discussion of the risk of failure. He says: "Those who have as their goal complete change of sexual orientation and who view failure to achieve a 'complete heterosexual shift' as evidence of lack of faith, lack of spiritual maturity, or as a sign of moral degradation may be in a far worse state than those who attempt change but recognize the potential limitations of change techniques. A related concern is that lack of success in treatment may lead to anger and resentment. These feelings may be directed inward (taking the form of depression or suicidality), or they may be directed at the therapist, family members, society, God, the church, support groups, and so on" (p. 256). Other conversion therapists frequently dismiss the possibility that they may have caused harm (cf. Dreifus, 1999; Nicolosi, 1999a).

CONCLUSION

Our study suggests that there are significant ethical issues in the application of sexual orientation conversion therapies. Interviews with consumers of conversion therapies indicate that many conversion therapists may not be practicing in a manner consistent with the APA Ethics Code (1992), similar professional codes by other mental health organizations, and guidelines on the appropriate treatment of gay and lesbian psychotherapy patients (Conger, 1975; ACA, 1999; APA, 1998, 2000; American Psychiatric Association, 2000).

It has been argued that any sexual orientation conversion treatment by a licensed mental health practitioner may be viewed as consumer fraud (Haldeman, 1991). According to these arguments, with the declassification of homosexuality as a mental disorder, the diagnosis of a homosexual orientation as a psychological disorder and subsequent interventions to treat it deceive the patient and the public that homosexuality is a pathological condition (Davison, 1991). Bryant Welch, former Executive Director of Practice Directorate of the American Psychological Association, stated in 1990 that "no scientific evidence exists to support the effectiveness of any of the conversion therapies that try to change one's sexual orientation" (as quoted in Herek, 2001). In Schreier's (1998) words, "The position . . . simply put, is: there is no illness, there is no cure" (p. 305). Many consumers reported to us that their conversion therapist did not inform them of the positions of the American Psychological Association and the American Psychiatric Association that scientific evidence demonstrates that a homosexual orientation is not associated with psychopathology.

This raises unsettling questions about the relationship between conversion therapists and the associations that determine the standards of practice for their profession. Nicolosi (2000), executive director of NARTH, has written a polemic entitled "Imagine . . ." in which he discusses the possibility of a class-action suit against the American Psychological Association and the American Psychiatric Association. Nicolosi justifies his adversarial position with the claim that the two APAs "*[fail] to disclose* that homosexuality is a treatable condition [italics in original]." He further argues that lesbians and gay men are not being "properly informed that acceptance of a gay identity would lead to greater risk for anxiety, depression, low self-esteem, loneliness, suicide attempts, failed relationships, drug use, alcohol abuse, tobacco use, and addiction to unhealthy (exotic) [sic] sexual practices, as well as STD'S [sic] and AIDS." Other conversion therapists feel that the American Psychological Association has "restricted the flow of information . . . necessary for science to function objectively" and "employed coercion to enforce its politics" and have called for the founding of a "Psychologists for a Free APA" group (Johnson, 1995, p. 53).

Based on interviews with consumers, we identified the following critical issues on the ethics of conversion therapies.

Informed Consent

In the area of informed consent we found several ethical lapses:

1. Clinicians did not provide accurate information about sexual orientation. Clients were told that a homosexual orientation is a psychological disorder or that it does not exist. Clinicians provided purportedly scientific, fraudulent information about gay lives and relationships which characterized them as unhappy and dysfunctional. Such statements do not reflect the current status of social scientific knowledge regarding the lived lives of gay men and lesbians. Conversion therapists who tell patients otherwise may be practicing unethically. As Singer (1980) has stated, in a paper on the scientific basis of psychotherapeutic practice, "The practitioner who has not examined recent developments in the research literature . . . may well be violating a central ethic of the profession" (p. 372).
2. Clinicians did not provide accurate information about the efficacy of the proposed intervention and prognosis. Many clients were told that high motivation and hard work in the treatment would assure a change in sexual orientation.
3. Alternative treatment options such as gay-affirmative therapy were only infrequently discussed.
4. Clinicians who were employed by religious universities may have a professional conflict of interest if they provide conversion therapy to students who are mandated to change their sexual orientation at the threat of academic expulsion.

Religion

A frank discussion and empirical research are needed about whether and when it is appropriate for a clinician to use religious justification for behavioral change or to threaten a client with religious consequences from a failure to change their sexual orientation. How do religious exhortations affect the practice of psychotherapy? When and how is it appropriate for the clinician to tell a patient about his own religious beliefs? What religious interventions are consistent with competent psychotherapy for lesbians and gay men who struggle with their sexual orientation? Richards and Potts (1995) have suggested that psychotherapists within each religious faith should develop ethical guidelines and standards of practice for clinicians who wish to use spiritual interventions. Although not writing about lesbians and gay men in psychotherapy, Bergin (1991, p. 399) has written a thoughtful statement on the issue of introducing religion into psychotherapy. He says:

> Although religious therapists often have a strong interest in value discussions, this can be problematic if it is overemphasized. It would be unethical to trample on the values of clients, and it would be unwise to focus on value issues when other issues may be at the nucleus of the disorder, which is frequently the case in the early stages of treatment. It is vital to be open about values but not coercive, to be a competent professional and not a missionary for a particular belief, and at the same time to be honest enough to recognize how one's value commitments may or may not promote health.

Pre-Termination Counseling

Proper pre-termination counseling with clients *who fail* conversion therapy appears to be especially neglected. Our respondents who failed to change sexual orientation indicated that they did not receive assistance from their conversion therapist in coming to terms with this failure or accepting a homosexual orientation. Clients not only blamed themselves for the failure to change, but were also sometimes blamed by their therapist. Furthermore, many conversion therapists do not appear to provide appropriate referrals for patients who failed to change.

Since a central component of conversion therapy is the indoctrination of patients with the belief that a homosexual orientation is a psychological disorder and is not compatible with a happy life and satisfying relationships (cf. Dallas, 1991; Moberly, 1983; Nicolosi, 1991, 1993; Satinover, 1996; Socarides, 1978, 1995), it is imperative that conversion therapy failures be provided with efficacious help to deal with the iatrogenically induced exacerbation of internalized homophobia.

Negative Side-Effects

In our view, informed consent has to include an accurate discussion of the possible negative effects of conversion therapy. Our research (Shidlo and Schroeder, 2001) suggests that many participants in sexual orientation conversion therapies are plagued by serious psychological and interpersonal problems after termination. These negative effects include depression, poor self-esteem, and difficulties with intimate relationships. These findings are consistent with the observations of others (American Psychiatric Association, 1998, 2000; Drescher, 2001b; Haldeman, 1991, 1994, 2001; Isay, 1990, 1997). Conversion therapists and their supporters have historically ignored the possible harm of their interventions. The recent recognition by Nicolosi et al. (2000) and Yarhouse (1998) of possible negative effects of conversion therapies represents a welcome shift.

How are we to understand the general neglect of negative effects in the conversion therapy literature? Research on negative outcomes in psychotherapy suggests that clients and therapists alike may have difficulties expressing and dealing with harm of treatment. Marsh and Hunsley (1993) have written that:

> Failures in therapy may also not be readily noted because they are sometimes hidden by the client, perhaps out of deference to authority, a desire to please the therapist, or the anticipation of therapist disapproval. Surprisingly, such client behavior may be adaptive, as most therapists have difficulty in recognizing and responding appropriately to negativity or critical feedback from clients (e.g., Colson, Lewis, and Horwitz, 1985; Hill, 1990). (p. 292)

Thus, one hypothesis for the neglect of negative effects in the conversion therapy literature is that clients may not be always telling their therapists about harm. Hill, Gelso, and Mohr (2000) have studied the complex phenomenon of client concealment and found that:

> Clients have reported keeping secrets because of feeling deferent toward therapists, feeling ashamed or embarrassed, not being able personally to handle the disclosure, thinking that the therapist could not handle the disclosure, being afraid to express feelings, being concerned that revealing secrets would show the therapist how little progress had been made, not having enough time, not being willing to tell anyone, not being motivated to address the secret, or feeling loyalty to someone else (Hill et al., 1993; Kelly, 1998; Rennie, 1994).

These findings are consistent with our data that many conversion therapy patients withheld from their therapists information about unchanged homosexual desire and behavior, as well as misrepresented the appearance of new heterosexual feelings (Shidlo and Schroeder, 2001). Many respondents told us that they left conversion therapy pretending to their therapist to have changed their sexual orientation. One participant said:

Toward the end, I just started acting, like going there and being all positive and happy; I still felt suicidal. Because I didn't know how to tell him I wanted to quit. I was afraid of him.

Conversion therapists need to assess and to attend to patients' concealed or unexpressed information about failure to change, desire to please, and fear of feeling blame. Process and outcome research on the long-term negative effects of conversion therapies are urgently needed.

NOTES

1. Hereinafter, this document is referred to as the APA Ethics Code.
2. Hereinafter this document is referred to as the APA's Resolution on Therapeutic Responses.
3. Hereinafter this document is referred to as the APA Guidelines for Psychotherapy.
4. Hereinafter this document is referred to as the Attempts to Change Sexual Orientation.
5. Promise Keepers (PK) describes itself as a "Christ-centered ministry dedicated to uniting men through vital relationships to become godly influences in their world." It has been termed a male supremacist group by the National Organization for Women (NOW) and, according to the Center for Democracy Studies, advances "the strategic political agenda of the Christian right." NOW reports that PK's leadership has been involved in anti-gay political activity (see www.promisekeepers.org, www.now.org/issues/right/pk.html, and www.cdsresearch.org/promise_keepers_watch.htm).

REFERENCES

ABC News. (1998, July 30). *Nightline.* Homosexuality, morality and politics: the political fate of homosexuality.

American Association for Marriage and Family Therapy. (1991). *AAMFT Code of Ethics.* Washington, DC: Author.

American Counseling Association. (1995). *Code of Ethics and Standards of Practice.* Alexandria, VA: Author.

American Counseling Association. (1999). *Discrimination Based on Sexual Orientation: History of the American Counseling Association's Position.* Alexandria, VA: Author.

American Psychiatric Association. (1998). *Position Statement on Psychiatric Treatment and Sexual Orientation* [On-line]. Available: <www.psych.org/news_stand/rep_therapy.cfm>.

American Psychiatric Association. (2000). *COPP Position Statement on Therapies Focused on Attempts to Change Sexual Orientation (Reparative or Conversion*

Therapies) [On-line]. Available: <www.psych.org/psych/htdocs/practof psych/ copptherapyaddendum83100.html>.

American Psychoanalytic Association. (2000). *Position Statement on Reparative Therapy* [On-line]. Available: <www.apsa- co.org/ctf/cgli/reparative_therapy.htm>.

American Psychological Association. (1992). *Ethical Principles of Psychologists and Code of Conduct*. Washington, DC: Author.

American Psychological Association. (1998). Appropriate therapeutic responses to sexual orientation in the proceedings of the American Psychological Association Incorporated, for legislative year 1997. *American Psychologist*, 53:882-939.

American Psychological Association. (2000). Guidelines for psychotherapy with lesbian, gay and bisexual clients. *American Psychologist*, 55:1440-1451.

Anderson, C.W., & Adley, A.R. (1997). *Gay and Lesbian Issues: Abstracts of the Psychological and Behavioral Literature, 1985-1996*. Washington, DC: American Psychological Association.

Bergin, A.E. (1991).Values and religious issues in psychotherapy and mental health. *American Psychologist*, 46:394-403.

Colson, D., Lewis, L., & Horwitz, L. (1985). Negative outcome in psychotherapy and psychoanalysis. In: *Negative Outcome in Psychotherapy and What to Do About It*, eds. D.T. Mays & C.M. Franks. New York: Springer, pp. 59-75.

Conger, J. (1975). Proceedings of the American Psychological Association for the year 1974: Minutes of the annual meeting of the Council of Representatives. *American Psychologist*, 30:620-651.

Dallas, J. (1991). *Desires in Conflict*. Eugene, OR: Harvest House Publishers.

Davison, G.C. (1991). Constructionism and morality in therapy for homosexuality. In: *Homosexuality: Research Implications for Public Policy*, eds. J.C. Gonsiorek & J.D. Weinrich. Newbury Park, NJ: Sage, pp. 137-148.

D'Augelli, A.R., & Patterson, C.J. (1995). *Lesbian and Gay Identities Over the Lifespan*. New York: Oxford University Press.

Dreifus, C. (1999, May 25). A conversation with John Bancroft: Sitting in the ultimate hot seat–The Kinsey Institute. *New York Times* [On-line]. Available: <www.nyt.com>.

Drescher, J. (2001a). I'm your handyman: A history of reparative therapies. *Journal of Gay & Lesbian Psychotherapy*, 5(3/4):5-24.

Drescher, J. (2001b). Ethical concerns raised when patients seek to change same-sex attractions. *Journal of Gay & Lesbian Psychotherapy*, 5(3/4):181-210.

Duberman, M. (1991). *Cures: A Gay Man's Odyssey*. New York: Dutton.

Flanagan, J.C. (1954). The critical incident technique. *Psychological Bulletin*, 51: 327-358.

Ford, J.G. (2001). Healing homosexuals: A psychologist's journey through the ex-gay movement and the pseudo science of reparative therapy. *Journal of Gay & Lesbian Psychotherapy*, 5(3/4):69-86.

Fraser, D. (1999). *QSR NUD*IST VIVO: Reference Guide (and Software)*. Melbourne, Australia: Qualitative Solutions and Research Pty. Ltd.

Garnets, L., Hancock, K.A., Cochran, S.D., Goodchilds, J., & Peplau, L.A. (1991). Issues in psychotherapy with lesbians and gay men. *American Psychologist*, 46: 964-972.

Gonsiorek, J.C. (1991). The empirical basis for the demise of the illness model of homosexuality. In: *Homosexuality: Research Implications for Public Policy,* eds. J.C. Gonsiorek & J.D. Weinrich. Newbury Park, NJ: Sage, pp. 101-114.

Haldeman, D.C. (1991). Sexual orientation conversion therapy for gay men and lesbians: A scientific examination. In: *Homosexuality: Research Implications for Public Policy,* eds. J.C. Gonsiorek & J.D. Weinrich. Newbury Park, NJ: Sage, pp. 149-160.

Haldeman, D.C. (1994). The practice and ethics of sexual orientation conversion therapy. *Journal of Consulting and Clinical Psychology,* 62:221-227.

Haldeman, D.C. (2001). Therapeutic antidotes: Helping gay and bisexual men recover from conversion therapies. *J. Gay & Lesbian Psychother.,* 5(3/4):117-130.

Herek, G. (2001). *Attempts to Change Sexual Orientation. Statement of Bryant L. Welch,* [On-line]. Available: <psychology.ucdavis.edu/rainbow/html/facts_changing. html>.

Hill, C.E. (1990). Exploratory in-session process research in individual psychotherapy: A review. *Journal of Consulting & Clinical Psychology,* 58:288-294.

Hill, C.E., Gelso, C.J., & Mohr, J.J. (2000). Client concealment and self-presentation in therapy: Comment on Kelly (2000). *Psychological Bulletin,* 126:495-500.

Hill, C.E., Thompson, B.J., Cogar, M.C., & Denman, D.W. (1993). Beneath the surface of long-term therapy: Therapist and client report of their own and each other's covert processes. *Journal of Counseling Psychology,* 40:278-287.

Isay, R. (1990). *Being Homosexual: Gay Men and Their Development.* New York: Morrow, William & Co.

Isay, R. (1997). *Becoming Gay: The Journey to Self-Acceptance.* New York: Pantheon.

Johnson, R.W. (1995). American psychology: The political science. *Collected Papers from the NARTH Annual Conference.* Encino, CA: National Association for the Research and Treatment of Homosexuality.

Kelly, A.E. (1998). Clients' secret keeping in outpatient therapy. *Journal of Counseling Psychology,* 45:50-57.

Kinsey, A.C., Pomeroy, W.B., & Martin, C.E. (1948). *Sexual Behavior in the Human Male.* Philadelphia: W.B. Saunders Company.

Liddle, B.J. (1999). Gay and lesbian clients' ratings of psychiatrists, psychologists, social workers, and counselors. *Journal of Gay & Lesbian Psychotherapy,* 3:81-93.

Martin, A.D. (1984). The emperor's new clothes: Modern attempts to change sexual orientation. In: *Innovations in Psychotherapy with Homosexuals,* eds. E.S. Hetrick & T.S. Stein. Washington, DC: American Psychiatric Press, pp. 23-57.

Marsh, E.J. & Hunsley, J. (1993). Assessment considerations in the identification of failing psychotherapy: Bringing the negatives out of the darkroom. *Psychological Assessment,* 5:292-301.

Miller, M. (2000, May 8). To be Gay–and Mormon. *Newsweek* [On-line]. Available: <www.newsweek.com>.

Moberly, E.R. (1983). *Homosexuality: A New Christian Ethic.* Cambridge, England: James Clarke & Company.

Moor, P. (2001). The view from Irving Bieber's couch: "Heads I win, tails you lose." *Journal of Gay & Lesbian Psychotherapy,* 5(3/4):25-36.

National Association for Research and Therapy of Homosexuality. (Undated document A). *Statement of policy.* [Brochure]. Encino, CA: Author.

National Association for Research and Therapy of Homosexuality. (Undated document B). *Taking a Stand for Those Seeking Freedom from Homosexuality* [Brochure]. Encino, CA: Author.

National Association of Social Workers. (1996). *Code of Ethics.* Washington, DC: Author.

Nicolosi, J. (1991). *Reparative Therapy of Male Homosexuality.* New Jersey: Jason Aronson Inc.

Nicolosi, J. (1993). *Healing Homosexuality: Case Stories of Reparative Therapy.* New York: Jason Aronson Inc.

Nicolosi, J. (1999a). *The Battle Against the APA Resolution* [On-line]. Available: <www.narth.com/docs/battleapa.html>.

Nicolosi, J. (1999b). Reflections from Jeffrey Satinover/NARTH Interviews Dr. Satinover. [On-line]. Available: <www.narth.com/reflections> from <jeffrey satinover.htm>.

Nicolosi, J. (2000). *Imagine . . .* [On-line]. Available: <www.narth.com/docs/imagine.html>.

Nystrom, N. (1997, February). *Mental Health Experiences of Gay Men and Lesbians.* Paper presented at the American Association for the Advancement of Science, Houston, Texas.

O'Neill, P.A. (1998). *Negotiating Consent in Psychotherapy.* New York: New York University Press.

Perez R.M., Debord K.A., & Bieschke, K.J. (2000). *Handbook of Counseling and Psychotherapy with Lesbian, Gay, and Bisexual Clients.* Washington, DC: American Psychological Association.

Pope, K.S., & Vetter, V.A. (1992). Ethical dilemmas encountered by members of the American Psychological Association: A national survey. *American Psychologist,* 47:397-411.

Rennie, D.L. (1994). Clients' deference in psychotherapy. *Journal of Counseling Psychology,* 41:427-437.

Rhodes, R.H., Hill, C.E., Thompson, B.J., & Elliott, R. (1994). Client retrospective recall of resolved and unresolved misunderstanding events. *Journal of Counseling Psychology,* 41:473-483.

Richards, P.S., & Potts, R.W. (1995). Using spiritual interventions in psychotherapy: Practices, successes, failures, and ethical concerns of Mormon psychotherapists. *Professional Psychology: Research & Practice,* 26:163-170.

Richards P.S., & Bergin A. E. (2000). *Handbook Of Psychotherapy and Religious Diversity.* Washington, DC: American Psychological Association.

Rubin, H.J, & Rubin, I.S. (1995). *Qualitative Interviewing: The Art of Hearing Data.* Thousand Oaks, CA: Sage.

Satinover, J. (1996). *Homosexuality and the Politics of Truth.* Grand Rapids, Michigan: Hamewith Books.

Schreier, B.A. (1998). Of shoes, ships, and sealing wax: The faulty and specious assumptions of sexual reorientation therapies. *Journal of Mental Health Counseling,* 20:305-314.

Shidlo, A., & Schroeder, M. (2001). *Conversion Therapy: A Consumers Report.* Unpublished manuscript.

Siegel, E.V. (1988). *Female Homosexuality: Choice with Volition*. Hillsdale, NJ: Lawrence Erlbaum.

Silverstein, C. (1977). Homosexuality and the ethics of behavioral intervention: Paper 2. *Journal of Homosexuality*, 2:205-211.

Singer, Jerome, L. (1980). The scientific basis of psychotherapeutic practice: A question of values and ethics. *Psychotherapy: Theory, Research & Practice*, 17: 372-383.

Socarides, C.W. (1978). *Homosexuality*. New York: Jason Aronson.

Socarides, C.W. (1995). *Homosexuality: A Freedom Too Far*. Phoenix, Arizona: Adam Margrave Books.

Stein, T.S. (1999), Commentary on Gay and lesbian clients' ratings of psychiatrists, psychologists, social workers, and counselors. *Journal of Gay & Lesbian Psychotherapy*, 3:95-100.

Throckmorton, W. (1998). Efforts to modify sexual orientation: A review of outcome literature and ethical issues. *Journal of Mental Health Counseling*, 20: 283-304.

van den Aardweg, G. (1997). *The Battle for Normality: A Guide for (Self-) Therapy for Homosexuality*. San Francisco, CA: Ignatius Press.

White, M. (1994). *Stranger at the Gate: To Be Gay and Christian in America*. New York: Simon & Schuster.

Yarhouse, M.A. (1998). When clients seek treatment for same-sex attraction: Ethical issues in the "right to choose" debate. *Psychotherapy*, 35:248-259.

Yarhouse, M.A., & VanOrman, B.T. (1999). When psychologists work with religious clients: Applications of the general principles of ethical conduct. *Professional Psychology: Research and Practice*, 30:557-562.

Yarhouse, M.A., & Burkett, L.A. (2000). *Respecting Religious Diversity: Possibilities and Pitfalls*. In M.A. Yarhouse (Chair), Gays, ex-gays, and ex-ex-gays: Examining key religious, ethical and diversity issues. Symposium conducted at the annual meeting of the American Psychological Association, Washington, DC, August 7, 2000.

Overview of Ethical and Research Issues in Sexual Orientation Therapy

Marshall Forstein, MD

SUMMARY. Attempts to change sexual orientation have evolved primarily out of moral and pathological beliefs about homosexuality, rather than out of neutral curiosity about the fluidity of human erotic desire. History is replete with violent examples of antihomosexual bias being purveyed in the guise of "medical cure" of what was considered a psychosexual arrested development. Research into the efficacy and desirability of changing sexual orientation has been marred by biased researchers and inadequate research principles and designs. Ethically, there are many questions raised concerning the behavior of therapists who try to change their patients' sexual orientation. Issues about research and ethical guidelines about therapy to change sexual orientation are addressed. *[Article copies available for a fee from The Haworth Document Delivery Service: 1-800-HAWORTH. E-mail address: <getinfo@haworthpressinc. com> Website: <http://www.HaworthPress.com> © 2001 by The Haworth Press, Inc. All rights reserved.]*

KEYWORDS. Conversion therapy, ethics, homosexuality, pathological view of homosexuality, psychotherapy, research, sexual orientation

Marshall Forstein is Assistant Professor of Psychiatry, Harvard Medical School at the Cambridge Hospital, and Medical Director, Mental Health and Addiction Services, Fenway Community Health Center.

This paper was presented at a Symposium entitled "Clinical Issues and Ethical Concerns Regarding Attempts to Change Sexual Orientation: An Update" at the annual meeting of the American Psychiatric Association in New Orleans, LA, May 9, 2001.

[Haworth co-indexing entry note]: "Overview of Ethical and Research Issues in Sexual Orientation Therapy." Forstein, Marshall. Co-published simultaneously in *Journal of Gay & Lesbian Psychotherapy* (The Haworth Medical Press, an imprint of The Haworth Press, Inc.) Vol. 5, No. 3/4, 2001, pp. 167-179; and: *Sexual Conversion Therapy: Ethical, Clinical and Research Perspectives* (ed: Ariel Shidlo, Michael Schroeder, and Jack Drescher) The Haworth Medical Press, an imprint of The Haworth Press, Inc., 2001, pp. 167-179. Single or multiple copies of this article are available for a fee from The Haworth Document Delivery Service [1-800-HAWORTH, 9:00 a.m. - 5:00 p.m. (EST). E-mail address: getinfo@haworthpressinc.com].

HISTORICAL PERSPECTIVE

Efforts to change sexual orientation with psychotherapy evolved primarily as a result of the medicalization of homosexuality and the increasing visibility of politically active homosexual individuals and organizations seeking greater acceptance in society. As with any political and cultural movement within the American society, such as the civil rights movement and women's liberation, countervailing forces have sprung up in opposition to the attempts to find accommodation of "outsiders" into positions of equality within the larger society.

Prior to the pathologizing of same-sex erotic and affectional desire in the modern age, homosexuality was viewed by society as a matter of moral sinfulness or antisocial behavior and homosexuality became the target of religious groups wishing to "heal" those afflicted with "moral degeneracy." With the advent of the medical view of psychosexual arrested development, psychoanalysts joined the movement to treat homosexuality. Buoyed by the association of femininity with male homosexuality, and the theories of unresolved oedipal issues, therapists rushed to the fore to promise that if early childhood problems were treated with intensive psychotherapy, that homosexuality could be "cured." This psychopathological view of homosexuality (particularly focused on male homosexuality) led to several theories of etiology without any scientific basis in research. The cultural acceptance of homosexuality as an illness pushed clinicians, therapists, doctors, and religious counselors to accept homosexuality as pathological without applying the same rigorous scientific principles as was expected in other fields of medicine.

Consequently, almost every branch of the biomedical and social sciences has been used to try to control sexual orientation. Efforts to change homosexual orientation to heterosexual have been made with every conceivable technology or psychological theory (Murphy, 1992). Attempts have included electroshock therapy after viewing graphic homoerotic pictures, convulsive therapy, nausea inducing drugs, testicular implants, behavior therapy and psychoanalysis (James, 1962). Biological attempts to change sexual orientation have included attempts to manipulate the sex hormones with the assumption that both men and women have homoerotic interests because they lack the appropriate gender hormone levels. Ironically, giving male hormones to homoerotically oriented men did not change their sexual orientation, but it did increase the intensity of their homoerotic interests. It is interesting to note that most attempts to cure or change homoerotic desire have faded into history–along with their proponents–while psychoanalytically informed approaches remain among the most durable attempts at "curing" homosexual orientation. Although the official position towards homosexuality of several psychoanalytic associations has changed, there remains a group of therapists who hold to the older psychoanalytic theoretical position that a homosexual orientation is, at best, an entrenched adaptation to the failure to achieve normative heterosexual orientation (Rado, 1940).

Much of the support for the movement to treat the "disorder" called homosexuality began with the 1952 classification by the American Psychiatric Association of homosexuality as a "sociopathic personality." Once this official pronouncement appeared, physicians, therapists and religious organizations began organizing programs to change those who appeared before them with distress about their homoerotic interests. The use of the diagnostic category of "sociopathic personality" played to the fears and anxieties that not only that certain types of sexual behavior were disordered, but inherently dangerous to society at large.

Today, right wing and fundamentalist religious organizations continue to characterize homosexuality as "a threat to society" or a threat to "family values." Using Biblical invectives against homosexuality (arguably misinterpreted–see Boswell, 1980), the religious and political right eschew science in the name of a "moral position." Perhaps more interesting to sociological researchers is the enormous fear that a small minority population (1-10%, depending on the study) could undermine the stability and value of traditional family configurations, as well as heterosexuality itself.

In 1968, the American Psychiatric Association declined to maintain the nomenclature "sociopathic personality," but continued to characterize homosexuality as a mental disorder. Only after much political action to bring data to the scientific body of the APA's workgroup on diagnoses was a discussion pursued to look at scientific studies that did not support the classification of homosexuality as a mental disorder. Psychologist Evelyn Hooker's famous 1957 study put to rest the notion that blinded and independent observers could ascertain homosexual orientation by psychometric testing. Along with the lack of any clear and convincing evidence that homosexually-oriented people fit criteria for a mental disorder, homosexuality was removed in 1973 from the *Diagnostic and Statistical Manual (DSM)* (Bayer, 1987). As it was acknowledged that some homosexually oriented people might have significant distress about their sexuality, the diagnostic category of "sexual orientation disturbance" was created, later replaced in 1980 by "ego dystonic homosexuality." This served to continue the movement to create opportunities for people to have their sexual orientation "changed" by therapists and religious organizations that continued to believe and promote the notion of homosexuality as a disorder, illness or moral weakness.

Although the APA removed "ego dystonic homosexuality" from the DSM in 1987, it retained a diagnostic category for treating people unhappy about their sexual orientation under "sexual disorders not otherwise specified." This continued pathologizing of homoerotic orientation was underscored by an

APA study in 1994 that showed most psychiatrists surveyed in Belarus, Brazil, China, India, Poland, Romania, Spain and Venezuela still considered homosexuality an illness (Van Hertum, 1994). By this time, all of the American mental health and medical professional associations had clearly issued policy statements declaring that homosexuality was *not* a mental disorder. Most recently, in April of 2001, the Chinese Psychiatric Society removed homosexuality as mental illness from its nomenclature.

So why, after the declassification of homosexuality as a mental disorder, is there still such controversy about whether sexual orientation can be changed? After all, regardless of the biomedical or psychological theory guiding the effort, the intention has been to increase heteroerotic interests in men and women and to suppress homoerotic interests. Rarely has there ever been an effort to *develop* or *enhance* homoerotic interests in either men or women. Not one of the groups or individuals supporting sexual orientation change therapy has supported that effort, making it clear that the efforts to change from hetero- to homoerotic is based on the underlying assumption that homosexuality per se is abnormal, undesirable, and problematic.

CURRENT STATE OF KNOWLEDGE

That some people may have changes in their erotic interests over the course of a lifetime does not provide evidence that, as a group, people with homoerotic interests can, or should, be treated to change those interests in a durable and psychologically integrative way. There is a fundamental difference between an individual's erotic interests changing over the life course, and an *intentional agenda on the part of any particular therapist* to change a particular person's erotic interests because of a fundamental belief that one erotic orientation is superior and psychologically preferable to another.

Murphy (1997) writes: "Currently, there is no confirmed method of altering the sexual orientation of people from the fundamental sexual interests, structures and patterns of interpersonal affection that they have as adults . . . There is no confirmed method of therapy that will fundamentally alter the sexual orientation of *randomly* selected men or women which are confirmably durable in regard to their erotic gender interests" (p. 82).

Who, in fact, are the people who would willingly choose to go to therapists who claim they can change a person's sexual orientation? What is the social, religious and psychological environment in which they grow up and then recognize homoerotic interests? Given the social mores and Judeo-Christian underpinnings of the American social structure, does the process of coming to terms with one's homoerotic interests *necessarily* imply a period of internalized fear and loathing of homoerotic interests (Shidlo, 1994)? A fundamental desire of all humans is to feel connection, to identify with others like oneself. Discovering one's sexual orientation to be homoerotic, and presumably different from one's family of origin and community, would require a rejection of one's own self in order to prevent the rejection by others who are assumed to be acceptable in the eyes of society. The psychiatric and psychological literature is replete with discussions about the need for peer identification as one part of the adolescent developing an independent self from that of the family (Hunter and Schaecher, 1987; Ramafedi, Farrow and Deisher, 1991). Adolescents who expect their homoerotic interests to alienate them from their peers often face a tremendous psychological stress and isolation in coming to terms with not identifying with peers, family or community. Is it possible to have a coherent, "normative" developmental view of sexual orientation independent of the social and cultural attitudes that stigmatize and marginalize non-heteroerotic interests?

RESEARCH CONCERNS

Research about the efficacy of therapy to change sexual orientation has been confused with questions concerning the etiology of homosexuality itself. While research that would explain the origins of any particular sexual orientation would not necessarily imply the need to change any such orientations, there are those who would use such data for the purpose of preventing homosexuality from arising as the dominant orientation in any particular individual. Failing to separate out the difference between furthering our understanding of the development of *all* orientations from the use of this understanding to promote one orientation over another contributes to the stigmatization of homoerotic interests (McKnight, 1997). *In the current climate of increasing visibility of homoerotically interested people–and the political issues of equal civil rights–I believe such scientific investigation must be undertaken with extreme caution, and with sensitivity to the potential misuse of science in the interests of social control over particular kinds of sexual behavior.*

There are several areas of interest that have been jumbled together, further confusing essential scientific and ethical questions. The first would be the research regarding the origins of any sexual orientation, and the relative contributions of genetics, embryological development and intrauterine experience, early childhood experience within and outside the family, and social and cultural influences. This research would have to start with a null hypothesis assuming no preferred outcome on the part of the researchers regarding the development of all sexual orientations, or otherwise the very construction of the necessarily complex research design to study these factors would be biased.

The second would be the construction of studies examining the underlying factors that separate those who would seek change from homoerotic to heteroerotic from those who more easily find acceptance of homoerotic orientation. Since we have found that suicidality is not uncommon among gay and lesbian teens and adults who are isolated, stigmatized, or unresolved about their sexual orientation (Schneider, Faberow and Kruks, 1989; Ramafedi, Farrow and Deisher, 1991), psychological and social variables would have to be studied to identify individuals for whom homosexual orientation is variably acceptable.

Thirdly, since people in distress about their sexual orientation find therapists willing and eager to help "cure" or change them, there is an interplay between who wants help changing and who wants to help. Given that the entire history of psychotherapeutic theory is built upon the very dynamic relationship between patient and therapist, this interplay must be understood in all of its complexity: the contribution of the psychological and social experience and beliefs of both patient and therapist.

Thus it would be incumbent on researchers to wonder as much about the question of desire to change erotic interests as a function of social stigma and individual fears and anxieties as they do about the possibility of such change over the long term. The National Institute of Mental Health Task Force on Homosexuality in 1972 concluded that psychological problems of gay people are primarily the function of social hostility and antihomosexual attitudes and beliefs within the major cultural and socially sanctioned structures. It further went on to say that there was no evidence that psychological problems are themselves derivative from the homoeroticism directly in the absence of the hostile social and political climate. Similarly, a 1994 report from the American Medical Association (published in 1996) stated that "much of the emotional disturbance experienced by gay men and lesbians around their sexual identity is not based on physiological causes but rather is due more to a sense of alienation in an unaccepting environment" (quoted in Murphy, 1997, p. 84).

Other important research challenges include the lack of agreed upon criteria for evaluating in a uniform manner those people who fall somewhere between an exclusive homo- or heteroerotic interest. There is currently not one prospective study with blinded observers to evaluate the outcome of therapies intended to change sexual orientation. There is no agreed upon classification system for categorizing the participants in such studies, nor is there consensus by any expert panel on the tools used to assess homoerotic and heteroerotic interests in a systematic manner. Consequently, there is no consistent method or criteria for either determining sexual orientation at the onset of therapy, nor any way to assess the durability or quality of such "change."

Research on the efficacy of therapy to change sexual orientation is problematic because the protocols to evaluate the starting point and stopping point of such therapy have not been subjected to peer review or reliability and validity studies. Sampling techniques to acquire subjects do not meet current standards of research. Not one study has been published to document the efficacy of a particular mode of therapy, nor has any theoretical basis for true change of erotic desire over the long term been described that is based on extensive clinical trials. Furthermore, there is no evidence that the therapy itself, rather than other forces or events, including the powerful wish to deny homoerotic interests and be "acceptable" as a "normal" member of society, is the causative modality for change.

Since there have been no objective screening criteria, no consensus about outcome measurement, and no blinded or side-by-side studies, all claims that there is any form of sexual orientation conversion therapy that is effective are without any scientific foundation. To date, not one peer reviewed research study, much less a prospective one that uses reliable and reproducible criteria, has been published in a respected peer reviewed scientific journal.

RESEARCH QUESTIONS

Many issues remain unclear in the absence of significant epidemiological, clinical or prospective research. Is sexual orientation fixed or fluid? If it can fluctuate during the life course of a particular individual, can it fluctuate in either direction? For whom and under what circumstances does it change? Is bisexuality somewhere between homoerotic and heteroerotic, or an entity unto itself? What percentage of the population experiences true shifts in sexual orientation over the life course as opposed to transient efforts to comply with social and religious expectations? Do men and women have similar or different determinants of shifting erotic interests? More fundamentally, why do people want to change their erotic interests? How would the motivation to change from homoerotic to heteroerotic be different in a culture in which one particular sexual orientation was no more valued than another? What are the psychodynamic issues that put particular individuals at risk for wanting to change homoerotic orientation to heteroerotic? What distinguishes those men and women who are comfortable with acknowledging their homosexuality from those who seek change?

ETHICAL ISSUES

There has been little discussion in the scientific literature about the ethics of sexual orientation therapy. Before the removal of homosexuality from the DSM as a disorder, it was assumed that psychoanalysis could treat the underlying "developmental disruption" and extinguish homoerotic desire. Even after homosexuality was no longer considered pathological, the discussion was centered on the etiology of sexual orientation and the rationale for trying to change homosexual to heterosexual, rather than the ethical issues of how such therapeutic interventions might occur or who might appropriately apply them in the clinical setting.

The question of the ethical nature of the practice of therapy to change sexual orientation has been raised in the political rather than scientific sphere, usually as a result of public gay protests. The ethical debate on the practice of psychotherapy to change sexual orientation has been conspicuously absent from the professional mental health literature. How is it that the scientific community has stood by almost silently and allowed professionals to report unproven practices without the critical scientific review that is applied to all other medical technologies? Murphy (1997), in his book *Gay Science* writes:

> Though no other efforts at reorientation were as collectively systematic and objectionable as those of Nazi Germany, condemnable reorientation efforts have transpired individually within the confines of private health care relationships around the world and in public institutions, sometimes at judicial order. The efforts to redirect sexual orientation may be in their historical totality just as objectionable as the historically transient but convulsive excesses of the Nazis. Many of the practices historically offered would today be summarily judged unethical not only because they violate ethical precepts in favor of informed consent and autonomous choice, but because they do not "fit" the "problem of homoeroticism." (p. 84)

ETHICAL PRECEPTS AND SEXUAL ORIENTATION CHANGE THERAPY

Religious organizations start with *a priori* assumptions that they are moral in their basic tenets. Nevertheless, they are not beyond legitimate discussion as to what constitutes ethical behavior of those organizations–or individuals within those organizations–in regard to attitudes and beliefs about homoerotically oriented people. It is beyond the scope of this paper to argue the purported Biblical basis for condemning homosexuality. It is, however, fair to ask the ethical question concerning the use of religious beliefs and organizational power by individuals acting *as therapists* to treat people in distress about their homoerotic desires. As a society we respect the right of religion to hold and teach such beliefs up until the point where those beliefs impinge on the very safety and integrity of the health of others. While we sanction the right to teach that life might start at conception, we do not sanction the violence towards those who support a woman's right to choose an abortion. We might tolerate religious beliefs about the need for marrying within one's own culture and religion, but we do not support the right for those beliefs to enact violence towards those who choose to bond inter-culturally or interracially. At each juncture, we have had to enact civil laws to protect those who are in the minority, or who do not hold political power, based on the ethical belief that it is wrong to hurt others on the basis of one's own particular beliefs. We still continue to see the conflict between religion and science in the battle between creationism and evolution.

More specifically, the ethics of the practice of psychotherapy have been developed as much out of the untoward effects of unethical therapists as by a basic set of ethical tenets. Yet of all the medical arts, psychotherapy has been less rigorously held to the basic tenets of ethical science and medicine. In fact, in some states, one can claim to be a "psychotherapist" even in the absence of any formal psychotherapy training.

I will not address in this paper the question of the ethics of pastoral or religious counselors, or of consumer self-help groups portraying themselves as able to change homosexual orientation. But for trained licensed psychotherapists there is a clear ethical responsibility to not confuse their personal religious or political beliefs with the science and practice of psychotherapy.

How then can we construct guidelines on how an ethical therapist might proceed with a patient who presents wanting to change their homosexual desire? What principles from the history of medicine might be borrowed to insure that both patient and therapist are on firm ethical grounds for proceeding with an inquiry into sexual orientation? It may be useful to reflect on how medical treatments in general have evolved along with both scientific and ethical guidelines.

Medical treatments fall into one of several categories. Most medical treatment derives from pathological states: infection leading to antibiotics, disruption of normal function leading to surgery, medications to enhance cardiac function, and so forth. These treatments derive from first identifying the underlying pathology, and then showing that the proposed treatment has a reasonable chance of improving quality of life, even if the disease process is not cured or stopped in its progression. The approval of treatments requires considerable study and review by peers who understand the pathology and are in a position to evaluate the risk/benefit ratio, and whether the treatment in question makes a statistically significant change in outcome. The degree of pathology and the risk for morbidity and mortality of not treating the underlying problem directly relates to the degree of significance expected for any given outcome. For example, whereas in the past vaccinations were deemed useful in forestalling epidemics only if they had a near 100 percent effectiveness, discussion now includes the use of an HIV vaccine that only approaches perhaps 30 percent. In the past this success rate would have been considered unacceptable. Given the impact that even a partially successful vaccine would make on the global AIDS epidemic, what may have been unethical in another situation is now on the table for discussion.

What drives these discussions on AIDS are as much ethical issues as scientific ones. Thus the seriousness of *not* treating a condition always needs to be weighed against the risks of treatment. The less essential the need for treatment in terms of psychological or physical health, the more rigorous must be the scrutiny of the treatment itself. If mortality rates from cosmetic plastic surgery were significantly higher than they are, the ethics of such treatment might well be brought into question. In the absence of empirical data that show clear and decisive benefit without risk of doing harm, how can treatments of a homosexual orientation, which is not a pathological condition, be sanctioned by society? Who decides what is reasonable risk? What are the roles of the consumer and the provider in this decision-making?

Such questions have led to certain agreed upon principles for medical treatments. When a new treatment is being considered, several questions must be asked and answered in order to follow traditional methodology for approval of new treatments:

1. What is the underlying condition being treated? Is the condition life threatening, or simply annoying? Is the condition based on biological pathology or social preferences?
2. What is the procedure for addressing the underlying condition? What basic science supports the treatment? In the absence of a basic scientific understanding of the treatment, are there other precepts or reliably consistent principles (like a reproducible psychological theory with research data behind it) that support a particular treatment? Have sufficient peer reviewed studies been conducted to support the particular intervention in question?
3. What are the risks and benefits of the proposed treatment? How were the risks and benefits assessed and communicated to the patient?
4. What population was studied and can the data be extrapolated to other populations?
5. What process was used to insure that the subject was indeed a "qualified subject," meaning did the condition being treated in all subjects have enough similarities to provide the evidence that the particular intervention was in itself responsible for the outcome and not by chance itself?

In light of the fact that a homosexual orientation has not been considered a psychologically pathological condition since 1973, ethically there would have to be a considerable burden to show that unproven treatments are clearly in the best interest of the patient. A useful analogy is that of cosmetic surgery, used not to correct an underlying medical condition, but to improve physical attributes because of the social pressure to enhance beauty, or to forestall the inevitable changes associated with aging. When a person presents requesting for cosmetic surgery, it is a standard of care to insure that the patient is aware of the risks and benefits, and to ascertain if there is an underlying psychological condition that would make even a good outcome insufficient or unacceptable to the patient. One would not, for instance, accede to performing surgery on someone who had a body dysmorphic disorder, for whom the particular surgical procedure would not be sufficient to resolve the underlying conflict over body image. While many people would harbor feelings that certain aspects of their bodies are less than what they would desire, body dysmorphic disorder can be a disabling condition which is not resolved by trying to appease the patient's wishes to physically change his body.

Similarly, given the social and religious disapprobation of homosexuality in society, it would be "normative" for a person who finds himself homoerotically driven to want to change that part of him to find acceptance and approval by families, and institutions, or even a supreme being. This alone would require a significant exploration by any ethical therapist as to the motivation in each particular case in which therapy to change from homoerotic to heteroerotic desire is sought. Thus, the essential question is whether in fact it is ever ethical for a therapist who believes that homosexuality is inferior to heterosexuality to engage in therapy with someone who is conflicted over sexual orientation.

To consider these issues, some basic guidelines for ethical practice may provide some clarification. When approached by a patient who wants to change their homosexual orientation, a therapist would employ these minimal standards of ethical practice. Any ethical intervention would at minimum include:

1. Informed consent that includes a statement of what the intervention is, on what it is based, and what the risks and/or benefits might be, including outcomes which could seriously hinder social, sexual, and psychological functioning. In all medical procedures it is expected that we inform patients of the statistical risk for any untoward potential event. These risk ratios are developed over years of studying the outcomes of particular procedures. It would be ethically necessary to inform the prospective patient that there are no studies as of yet published in peer reviewed, scientific, respected journals to provide these data. It would be incumbent on the therapist to provide a written statement to the effect of: "while it might be possible to increase heterosocial comfort and enhance whatever heterosexual interests might already exist, there is no evidence that therapy of any kind can induce new, sustainable heteroerotic interests in someone with a significant homoerotic orientation."

2. A clear and comprehensible statement of the current level of knowledge and the scientific basis for the intervention. This would include a clear acknowledgement that the therapist is engaging in a modality of treatment that is not considered appropriate to the situation for which the patient presents. This would require providing written policies and guidelines from the professional organization appropriate to the professional discipline of the practitioner. A clear statement that all U.S. mental health associations do not consider homosexual orientation to be a disorder must be provided to the patient.
3. Patients should know the status of the practitioner's standing in the professional community and with relevant licensing entities.
4. Therapists who have a clear belief system that finds homosexuality unacceptable must make it clear that they hold such beliefs.
5. Therapists who hold such beliefs and claim to be able to help the patient change sexual orientation would ethically be required to encourage a second opinion from a therapist who holds to the positions of the major mental health associations that officially designate sexual orientation conversion therapy to be outside the bounds of ethical, clinical standards of care.

Therapists ultimately have a fiduciary responsibility to their patients, to put the best interest of the patient above all, and to do no harm. While therapists hold all sorts of values that might differ from their patients, they carry the responsibility to investigate whatever underlying motivations and conflicts the patient brings, exploring without judgment or shaming the patient. Powerful transferences and countertransferences arise in any therapy, but where patients feel the disapproval of family, society and often even God, therapists have an even more profound obligation to not support self-negating or self-loathing feelings which accompany the wish to change from homosexual to heterosexual. For any therapist to have a particular agenda to change someone's sexual orientation undermines the essential ethical requirement to, above all else, put their own beliefs and those of the church and state secondary to the needs of their patient. Since homosexuality is not a pathological psychological disorder, therapists must first help patients to understand why they feel the way they do, without promulgating a particular belief that such feelings are wrong and changeable.

When a patient goes to a therapist who supports the pathological notion of homoerotic orientation, and who then claims to be able to alter that orientation through intensive therapy, the process is ethically compromised from the beginning. Indeed, in the treatment of individuals conflicted over their homosexual orientation, perhaps the only ethical situation would be one in which the therapist does not believe that it is necessary to change sexual orientation to find happiness, intimacy or love.

REFERENCES

American Psychiatric Association (1952), *Diagnostic and Statistical Manual of Mental Disorders*. Washington, DC: American Psychiatric Association.
American Psychiatric Association (1968), *Diagnostic and Statistical Manual of Mental Disorders, 2nd Edition*. Washington, DC: American Psychiatric Press.
American Psychiatric Association (1980), *Diagnostic and Statistical Manual of Mental Disorders, 3rd Edition*. Washington, DC: American Psychiatric Press.
American Psychiatric Association (1987), *Diagnostic and Statistical Manual of Mental Disorders, 3rd Edition–Revised*. Washington, DC: American Psychiatric Press.
American Psychiatric Association (1994), *Diagnostic and Statistical Manual of Mental Disorders, 4th Edition*. Washington, DC: American Psychiatric Press.
Bayer, R. (1987), *Homosexuality and American Psychiatry: The Politics of Diagnosis*. Princeton, NJ: Princeton University Press.
Boswell, J. (1980), *Christianity, Social Tolerance and Homosexuality*. Chicago, IL: University of Chicago Press.
Council on Scientific Affairs, American Medical Association (1996), Health care needs of gay men and lesbians in the United States. *JAMA*, 275(17):1354-1359.
Hooker, E. (1957), The adjustment of the male overt homosexual. *J. Proj. Tech*, 21:18-31.
Hunter, J. & Schaecher, R. (1987), Stresses on lesbian and gay adolescents in schools. *Social Work in Education*, 9(3), 180-190.
James, B. (1962), A case of homosexuality treated by aversion therapy. *Brit. Med. J.*, 1:768-770.
McKnight, J. (1997), *Straight Science? Homosexuality, Evolution and Adaptation*. London: Routledge.
Murphy, T. F. (1992), Redirecting sexual orientation: Techniques and justifications. *J. Sex Research*, 29:501-523.
Murphy T. F. (1997), *Gay Science: The Ethics of Sexual Orientation Research*. New York: Columbia University Press.
National Institute of Mental Health Task Force on Homosexuality (1972), *Final Report and Background Papers*. Department of Health, Education and Welfare: Washington, DC.
Rado, S. (1940), A critical examination of the concept of bisexuality. *Psychosomatic Medicine*, 2:459-467. Reprinted in *Sexual Inversion: The Multiple Roots of Homosexuality*, ed. J. Marmor. New York: Basic Books, 1965, pp. 175-189.
Remafedi, G., Farrow, J. A. & Deisher, R. W. (1991), Risk factors for attempted suicide in gay and bisexual youth. *Pediatrics*, 87(6):869-875.
Shidlo, A. (1994), Internalized homophobia: Conceptual and empirical issues in measurement. In: *Lesbian and Gay Psychology: Theory, Research, and Clinical Applications*, B. Greene & G. M. Herek, eds. Thousand Oaks: CA: Sage, pp. 176-205.
Schneider, S. G., Farberow, N. L. & Kruks, G. N. (1989), Suicidal behavior in adolescent and young adult gay men. *Suicide & Life Threat. Behav.*, 19(4) 381-394.
Van Hertum, A. (1994), Many psychiatrists still see homosexuality as an illness. *Washington Blade*, 24(40):31.

Ethical Concerns Raised
When Patients Seek
to Change Same-Sex Attractions

Jack Drescher, MD

SUMMARY. Since the American Psychiatric Association removed homosexuality from its diagnostic manual in 1973, mainstream mental health organizations have maintained that an individual's sexual orientation should be respected. Reparative therapists, however, argue that homosexuality is always a symptom of mental illness which should be treated. They have further argued that all therapists have an ethical responsibility to refer individuals with antihomosexual religious beliefs to reparative therapists in order to change their sexual identities.

This paper argues that such recommendations are unwise because they are derived from a misleadingly narrow reading of ethical guidelines. Rather than an issue regarding ethical patient care, this argument is a reflection of the culture wars surrounding homosexuality. This paper places those struggles in historical context. It examines reparative therapists' pathologizing of and attempts to "cure" or change same sex attractions. Reparative therapists insist on social and traditional gender conformity as a therapeutic goal, and in doing so operate from an essentialist

Jack Drescher is Training and Supervising Analyst at the William Alanson White Psychoanalytic Institute; Editor-in-Chief of the *Journal of Gay & Lesbian Psychotherapy* and author of *Psychoanalytic Therapy and the Gay Man* (The Analytic Press); Immediate Past President of the New York County District Branch of the APA and a member of its Committee on Ethics. Dr. Drescher is in private practice in New York City.

Address correspondence to: Jack Drescher, 420 West 23rd Street, #7D, New York, NY 10011 (E-mail: jadres@psychoanalysis.net).

[Haworth co-indexing entry note]: "Ethical Concerns Raised When Patients Seek to Change Same-Sex Attractions." Drescher, Jack. Co-published simultaneously in *Journal of Gay & Lesbian Psychotherapy* (The Haworth Medical Press, an imprint of The Haworth Press, Inc.) Vol. 5, No. 3/4, 2001, pp. 181-210; and: *Sexual Conversion Therapy: Ethical, Clinical and Research Perspectives* (ed: Ariel Shidlo, Michael Schroeder, and Jack Drescher) The Haworth Medical Press, an imprint of The Haworth Press, Inc., 2001, pp. 181-210. Single or multiple copies of this article are available for a fee from The Haworth Document Delivery Service [1-800-HAWORTH, 9:00 a.m. - 5:00 p.m. (EST). E-mail address: getinfo@haworthpressinc.com].

181

view of antihomosexual morality. Reparative therapies rely upon gender stereotyping that disrespects a patient's same-sex attractions. Furthermore, as some reparative therapists actively support political activities opposed to granting civil rights to lesbians and gay men, these activities raise ethical issues relevant to the entire psychotherapeutic endeavor. Inevitably, the decision about what social status to accord homosexuality is a moral and ethical issue affecting all patients and clinicians. *[Article copies available for a fee from The Haworth Document Delivery Service: 1-800-342-9678. E-mail address: <getinfo@haworthpressinc.com> Website: <http://www.HaworthPress.com> © 2001 by The Haworth Press, Inc. All rights reserved.]*

KEYWORDS. Antihomosexual bias, culture wars, ethical issues, gay and lesbian patients, gender stereotyping, homosexuality, psychiatric ethics, psychotherapy, reparative therapy, respect for patients, sexual conversion therapy

A physician shall be dedicated to providing competent medical service with compassion and respect for human dignity.

Principles of Medical Ethics of the American Medical Association[1]

In a recent paper (Yarhouse, 1988), it has been argued that psychologists, and presumably other therapists as well, have "an ethical responsibility to allow individuals to pursue treatment aimed at curbing experiences of same-sex attraction or modifying same-sex behaviors" (p. 248). The putative basis for this responsibility is the author's novel interpretation of the American Psychological Association's ethical principles (1992), particularly Section D, which urges therapists to give "respect to the fundamental rights, dignity, and worth of all people" (p. 1599) and a client's right to "privacy, confidentiality, self-determination, and autonomy" (p. 1600). This latter principle, according to the author, means patients or clients should have "a right to choose" psychotherapies designed to change their sexual feelings. He further argues that there are individuals whose religious beliefs require them to abandon their same-sex desires and to avoid homosexual behaviors. In other words, if a patient's religious beliefs are unaccepting of homosexuality, a therapist's respect for those beliefs justifies helping the patient rid him or herself of same-sex attractions.

Significant and troubling difficulties would arise in accepting such an interpretation of ethical principles. In the first place, it is an approach which is antithetical to psychotherapy treatments which are based on a model of intrapsychic conflict. Furthermore, how would one apply this principle to analogous religious conflicts? For example, what ethical principles should

guide the therapist treating a patient whose beliefs prohibited religious inter-
marriage? If that patient became involved with someone of another faith,
would respect for the patient's religion ethically oblige a therapist to automati-
cally choose to help the patient terminate his or her religiously forbidden relationship?[2]

A second, related problem to this author's argument is its overly narrow approach to the complexity of ethics and ethical reasoning. In most instances,
clinical ethical principles are usually intended to provide guidelines, rather
than definitive rules to resolve problematic situations. The interpretation of an
ethical principle is not equivalent to a fundamentalist reading of the bible.
Only by weighing potentially conflicting principles can one ultimately arrive
at a reasoned ethical decision. From a clinically ethical perspective, and in
keeping with standards of contemporary psychoanalytic practice, one must not
only respect the patient's wish to change, one must also respect the depth and
intensity of the patient's homosexual feelings and the wish to act on them. It is
only after such a process has ensued that a patient can possibly come to terms
with his or her own contradictory wishes and feelings. In the reparative therapy
literature, however, the only alternative to sexual orientation conversions for a
patient unhappy about his or her homosexuality is celibacy (Harvey, 1987;
Nicolosi, 1991).

What motivates this appeal for narrow ethical guidelines? It is a broader
agenda, one which interweaves clinical issues and politics, particularly as they
relate to the proper "treatment" of homosexuality. The political nature of this
issue has been addressed in professional journals (Blechner, 1993; Lesser,
1993; Schwartz, 1993; Trop and Stolorow, 1993; MacIntosh, 1994; Friedman
and Downey, 1995). Today, however, the reparative therapy debate has moved
out of the professional arena and into the cultural one. It has included advertisements in major newspapers promoting religious "cures" for homosexuality
(Dreyfuss, 1999) and exhortations, like the following, on the op-ed page of the
Wall Street Journal: "If a therapist feels for whatever reason that he cannot
treat someone for this [homosexual] condition, he has an obligation to refer the
patient to someone who will" (Socarides et al., 1997).

This paper argues that any putative ethical obligation to refer a patient for
reparative therapy is outweighed by a stronger ethical obligation to keep patients away from mental health practitioners who engage in questionable clinical
practices. To help clinicians better understand the sociopolitical and clinical
issues of this debate, this paper will attempt to place the "culture wars" surrounding homosexuality in a historical context. It examines reparative therapists' pathologizing of and attempts to "cure" or change same sex attractions.
Although reparative therapists maintain that sexual conversion therapies have
met rigorous, scientific standards of efficacy, that is not the case. This paper
will illustrate how reparative therapists instead rely upon gender stereotyping
in their clinical work and denigrate a patient's same-sex attractions. This paper

further outlines how reparative therapists insist on social and traditional gender conformity as a therapeutic goal, and work within what could be called an essentialist view of antihomosexual morality. Because some reparative therapists publicly participate in antigay political activities, their behaviors raise ethical issues relevant to the entire psychotherapeutic endeavor.

HISTORICAL PERSPECTIVE

Although same-sex attractions and behaviors have existed for millennia, the term "homosexuality" did not exist before the 19th century (Bullough, 1979; Greenberg, 1988; Katz, 1995). In that era, the medicalization of same-sex feelings and behaviors, by labeling them as "disease," was part of a new and enlightened tradition. In what Szasz (1974) refers to as the transition from the Religious State to the Therapeutic State, social phenomena such as alcohol use, unconventional sexual behaviors and insanity were reconceptualized in a scientific, medical model rather than in a religious one.

In the 19th and early 20th century, these nosological changes were considered triumphs of reason and progress over religious superstition. As an alternative to condemning sinners, the medical community held that it was not a person's fault if they were sick; those who were ill needed a physician's care and help, rather than punishment. Just as drunkenness became alcoholism, the Religious State's sin of sodomy became the Therapeutic State's disease of homosexuality. Not surprisingly, the medical model appealed to many individuals with same-sex feelings who welcomed the designation of "illness" over that of "sinner."

Freud (1935) wrote that "Homosexuality is assuredly no advantage, but it is nothing to be ashamed of, no vice, no degradation; it cannot be classified as an illness; we consider it to be a variation of the sexual function, produced by a certain arrest of sexual development" (p. 423).[3] Nevertheless, later psychodynamic theorists took a different tack. They regarded homosexuality as a difficult psychopathological problem which required modifications of traditional therapeutic neutrality (Eissler, 1953; cf. Lewes, 1988). Martin Duberman's account of his own treatment was typical of psychoanalytic approaches during a period when homosexuality was believed by clinicians to be a phobic avoidance of the other sex:

> From the first, [Duberman's psychiatrist] Weintraupt advised me to give up the relationship with [his lover] Larry. Until I did, he warned, any real progress in therapy would prove impossible. The drama of our interpsychic struggle, Weintraupt insisted, had become a stand-in for the more basic intrapsychic conflict I was unwilling to engage–the conflict between my neurotic homosexual "acting out" and my underlying healthy impulse toward a heterosexual union.

I resisted–not so much Weintraupt's theories, as his insistence on a total break with Larry. I accepted the need, but could not summon the will. I spent therapy hour after therapy hour arguing my inability to give up the satisfactions of the relationship–neurotic and occasional though they might be, and though my future happiness might well hang on their surrender. I resisted so hard and long that Weintraupt finally gave me an ultimatum: either give up Larry or give up therapy. (Duberman, 1991, p. 33)

Sandor Rado was the individual most influential in redefining homosexuality as a sign of pathological development (1940, 1969). He had a major influence on the work of Bieber (Bieber et al., 1962), Socarides (1968, 1978, 1995), Ovesey (1969), Hatterer (1970) and Siegel (1988). An offshoot of his theory can also be found in a fusion of religious and psychoanalytic approaches (Moberly, 1983; Nicolosi, 1991) which coined the term, "reparative therapy." The latter has increasingly come to generically define talking cures that try to change a person's homosexual identity to a heterosexual one. Despite claims of efficacy, however, the low conversion rates, 27-35% (Bieber et al., 1962; Socarides, 1995), are not particularly encouraging. Furthermore, the long-term effects of these treatments have not been well studied (Haldeman, 1991), although a study of several hundred patients is currently in progress (M. Schroder and A. Shidlo, in this volume). That is why the American Psychiatric Association (1998)[4] has issued a position statement that opposes any type of reparative therapy based upon the *a priori* assumption that homosexuality *per se* is an illness (Zwillich, 1999). In 2000, the American Psychiatric Association expanded upon that earlier statement, and has called into question the ethics of practitioners offering that treatment modality.[5]

HOMOSEXUALITY AND THE CULTURE WARS

On the surface, arguments about homosexuality can be viewed as a legitimate disagreement between scientists and clinicians. On one side is the reparative therapy perspective: Heterosexuality is the normal, expected outcome of development and homosexuality always represents a response to traumatic, environmental stimuli. This means that adult homosexuality can never be considered normal since it is always caused by psychological trauma in the early years of life. In this model, families usually bear the responsibility for damaging the future homosexual child. The most common culprits in these narratives are mothers, although fathers often get their share of blame. In addition, homosexuality is believed to be always accompanied by other psychopathology, presumably in the borderline or psychotic range of personality structure (Socarides, 1978). Psychotherapeutic treatments aim for a "normative" heterosexual adaptation, but are only possible if the "homosexual person" is sufficiently motivated to change. Anything other than a heterosexual outcome is considered suboptimal. Finally, reparative therapists consider social opprobrium of homosexuality to be an essential part of their treatment approach. Depending on the theorist, societal expressions of antihomosexuality, such as sodomy laws which criminalize same-sex activities, are regarded as a necessary part of human evolutionary design (Socarides, 1994b) or as consistent with the will of a higher power (Moberly, 1983).

On the other side of this issue are clinicians, as well as scientists, scholars and researchers in biology, biochemistry, endocrinology, ethology, evolutionary studies, experimental psychology, genetics, history, literary theory, neuroanatomy, the social sciences, and philosophy who offer an alternative understanding of homosexuality (Kinsey et al., 1948; Ford and Beach, 1951; Kinsey et al., 1953; Hooker, 1957; Marmor, 1965, 1980; Bell, Weinberg, and Hammersmith, 1981; McWhirter, Sandersm, and Reinisch, 1990; DeCecco and Parker, 1995). A growing body of research offered compelling evidence that homosexuality was not always associated with psychopathology and, as a result, a scientific hypothesis gained ground which maintained that same-sex attractions were a normal variant of human sexuality. It was this body of evidence which led the American Psychiatric Association (APA) to delete homosexuality *per se* from its official diagnostic nomenclature in 1973.

That act was a controversial decision (Bayer, 1981). At the time, some psychiatrists responded to the decision as an attack upon their own theories and practices. They, in turn, challenged the APA decision and called for a public referendum by the organization's membership. Even though a majority of APA members voted to uphold the diagnostic change, that still did not settle what was to become an ongoing, vituperative controversy fueled by the losing side. One opponent of the APA decision later argued in a psychiatric textbook that "Truth cannot be determined by vote, even by supposed authorities" (Gadpaille, 1989, p. 1087). Another accused the APA of miscounting the votes (Socarides, 1995, p. 179) and labeled the Chair of APA's Committee on Nomenclature, which authorized the change, "someone who crosses far over the line, from science to open advocacy of a political position" (p. 166).

In a cogent political analysis of the events surrounding the 1973 decision, Bayer (1981) argued that "The status of homosexuality is a political question, representing a historically rooted, socially determined choice regarding the ends of human sexuality" (p. 5). Bayer was pessimistic about the APA's ability to elevate the denigrated social status of homosexuality. He contended that "the psychiatric mainstream must ultimately affirm the standards of health and disease of the society within which it works. It cannot hold to discordant views regarding the normal and abnormal, the desirable and undesirable, and continue to perform its socially sanctioned function" (p. 194). However Bayer's conclusions, published only eight years after that event, were in error. The years since homosexuality was depathologized have been characterized by an unprecedented social acceptance of gay men and women in both public and private arenas.[6] Even psychoanalytic organizations that objected to the 1973 APA decision are now actively recruiting and training lesbian and gay candidates (Roughton, 1995).

Many of these changes which have taken place in the past decade can be attributed to the fact that depathologizing homosexuality denied religious, political, governmental, military, media, and educational institutions (medical or scientific) cover for rationalizing discrimination. As a result, the often-rancorous debates surrounding homosexuality have shifted from medical and scientific arenas to the social and political forums where they more properly belong. In the wider world, these social, political, and moral struggles have been referred to as the "culture wars" (Dreyfuss, 1999).

Without medical, psychological and psychiatric cover, contemporary discussions of the legal and social status of lesbians and gay men have brought to the surface many previously inarticulated, although culturally diffuse, anti-homosexual beliefs. Some segments of modern society have expressed a hostile rejection of homosexuality and consider it an unacceptable form of social expression. While some of the opposition is secular, as in the military high command, much of it is religious. However, the antihomosexual camp has modified its position somewhat in recent years. Many religious denominations have recently begun to espouse a philosophy of "loving the homosexual sinner while hating the sin of homosexuality." That is to say, they no longer regard homosexual thoughts and feelings to be equivalent to sinful homosexual deeds. As part of this evolution, some religious institutions are energetically attempting to resuscitate the 19th century's illness model of homosexuality (Dreyfuss, 1999). As mainstream mental health professions promote increased tolerance and acceptance of same-sex feelings, behaviors and relationships, they have had to contend with opposition from those who fervently opposed the societal normalization of homosexuality. Mental health organizations have been inexorably drawn into the culture wars; they are simultaneously being courted as allies in the fight for gay and lesbian civil rights by one side and demonized as pawns of the "homosexual agenda" by the other. As a consequence, it has become difficult, if not impossible, for today's clinicians to hide their own feelings on this issue behind a screen of either political or therapeutic neutrality.

REPARATIVE THERAPISTS AS POLITICAL ACTIVISTS

With the American Psychological Association, the American Psychiatric Association, the National Association of Social Workers, and the American

Psychoanalytic Association now endorsing a normal variant model of homo-sexuality, reparative therapists formed their own organization: The National Association for Research and Therapy of Homosexuality (NARTH). NARTH provides a politically conservative, counter-cultural base for those clinicians who disagree with the mainstream's acceptance of homosexuality.

Consistent with its position on the antihomosexual side of the culture wars, NARTH has also adopted an attitude of "love the sinner but hate the sin." In fact, although they espouse an antihomosexual treatment philosophy, repara-tive therapists paradoxically claim to be defenders of "homosexuals." The fol-lowing is typical of their claims: "The homosexual must be granted freedom from persecutory laws as well as full civil rights–and this constitutes an inte-gral part of our approach to homosexual individuals. . . . [yet] while we ask for civil rights, we also ask for the legitimate psychiatric rights of homosexuals to seek help for what they correctly feel is a disorder" (Socarides, 1994a). It should be noted, however, that the only gay civil right that the reparative ther-apy movement actively promotes is the right to undergo reparative therapy. Despite their claims of support for civil rights, reparative therapists have filed affidavits in support of Colorado's antigay Amendment Two (Socarides, 1993). That state law, which was eventually overturned by the Supreme Court, would have prevented any local municipality from offering civil rights pro-tections to lesbians and gay men (Greenhouse, 1996). Reparative therapists also supported unsuccessful defenses of sodomy laws in Tennessee (*Campbell v. Sundquist*) in 1995 and Louisiana (Cohen, 1998a, b) in 1998. These actions are consistent with a belief that the social opprobrium of homosexuality must be maintained and reinforced if heterosexuality is to be socially privileged. As one prominent reparative therapist put it, when challenged about these politi-cal activities: "Legal cases now in the courts do not concern whether gays should be stripped of their civil rights or should have them. . . . We believe harm would be done if our laws were to affirm homosexuality as indistinguish-able from heterosexuality. . . . We believe it is NARTH's responsibility to counter gay-activist testimony with our perspective, which gay activists call 'heterosexist,' but which has long served as a foundation of Western civiliza-tion and cannot be discarded with mere impunity" (Nicolosi, 2000).[7]

In pursuit of that agenda, reparative therapists have demonstrated a willing-ness to ally themselves with religious denominations that condemn homosexual-ity. Thus, a recent paid newspaper advertisement by the New Hampshire Christian Coalition cites a NARTH claim that same-sex couples are unstable (New Hampshire Christian Coalition, 1999).[8] Both the ad and the NARTH re-port are part of a concerted political effort to deny adoption rights to lesbians and gay parents and is part of a general alignment of the reparative therapy move-ment with socially conservative, antihomosexual religious groups. Ironically, some of these groups are not entirely comfortable with scriptural interpretation alone in justifying their antihomosexual morality. In the same way they use creation scientists to challenge conventional scientific wisdom (Tiffen, 1994), these groups seek scientific rationalizations to justify their positions. Reparative therapists have been willing to serve as their antihomosexual mental health experts (Dreyfuss, 1999). In doing so, even the scientific debates regarding the presumed etiologies of homosexuality have been subsumed within the culture wars.

REPARATIVE THERAPY:
AN ESSENTIALIST VIEW OF ANTIHOMOSEXUAL MORALITY

Many arguments have emerged in the nature/nurture debate surrounding homosexuality, a debate which has not yet been resolved to anyone's satisfaction (DeCecco and Parker, 1995). Modern sexology appears to be moving toward an interactionist view which acknowledges both biological and cultural contributions. Reparative therapists, on the other hand, adamantly refute essentialist claims that people are "born gay" and reject the argument that individuals with same-sex feelings should be helped to become more comfortable with them. Yarhouse (1998), for example, criticizes what he calls the "gay-affirmative" therapeutic stance for drawing upon unproven essentialist arguments regarding the origins of homosexuality.[9] In a similar vein, Nicolosi (1991) argues that "Scientific evidence has confirmed that genetic and hormonal factors do not seem to play a determining role in homosexuality. However, there continue to be attempts to prove that genetics rather than family factors determines homosexuality. These continuing efforts reflect the persistence of gay advocates to formulate a means by which homosexual behavior may be viewed as normal" (p. 87).

Others (Byne and Stein, 1997) have convincingly argued that respect for homosexuality should not depend upon an essentialist view of its presumed "etiology." Even in the unlikely event that people "choose" to be gay, such a choice could be respected in the way that one respects an individual's choice of religion or political party. However, the antihomosexual argument in the culture wars is that if one is not born gay, then same-sex attractions should not be respected. Even those who concede that homosexuality might be intrinsic compare it to the genetic trait of alcoholism. Although the latter may also be part of the natural order, its behavioral expression must be controlled to maintain social order.

In some cases, the political skirmishes surrounding etiological theories have achieved the status of dogma on both sides of the culture wars. Each side rhetorically elevates some presumably essential aspect of human identity as requiring protection from harmful environmental influences. On one side, "essentially gay" people are seen as needing protection from cultural homophobia. On the other, homosexually-oriented individuals with an "essential antihomosexual morality" must not fall victim to a "pro-gay agenda."

The prototype for these arguments can be found in the work of George Weinberg (1972), who is generally credited with coining the term *homophobia*. His formulation transposed the medical model of homosexuality in a novel way: He started with the premise that homosexuality is essentially normal. Consequently, same-sex attractions were not a sign of mental illness, but intolerance of homosexuality was considered one instead.[10] His perspective demonstrates how a 20th-century theorist can construct a clinical syndrome called homophobia in much the same way that 19th-century scientists created a disease called homosexuality (Greenberg, 1988; Katz, 1995).

Weinberg's contribution to the reparative therapy debate is seen in the routine denials of homophobia and bigotry that are now part of the usual discourse by reparative therapists. Consider Nicolosi's (1991) contention that "many who use the term [homophobia] neglect to acknowledge that without being 'phobic' about it, it is quite possible to reject the gay life-style within the framework of one's own values . . . it is simply a nonacceptance of the [gay] life-style as a viable and natural alternative" (p. 138). This kind of assertion was unheard of in an earlier era, when curing homosexuality was characterized as a purely medical or scientific endeavor. Nicolosi, however, argues that he does not suffer from a psychiatric disorder called "homophobia." Instead, he believes his attitudes are expressions of his innate self and values. He refutes his homophobia, although not his antihomosexuality, by adopting a position that parallels the beliefs of gay men who also declare that they do not suffer from an illness, "homosexuality," but that they are only expressing their own values, or their true selves.

The reparative therapy movement has taken the position that if an individual believes his homosexuality is wrong, that is sufficient to justify psychotherapeutic attempts to change it. They treat an individual's antihomosexual morality as an integral part of a person's character. However, because they regard antihomosexual moral values as essential, reparative therapists act as if respect for a patient's religious beliefs means unquestioning agreement with them. This is a clinical position with therapeutically troubling implications. At the present time, many religious denominations are wrestling with both normalizing (Boswell, 1980, 1994; Carrol, 1997; Gomes, 1996; Helminiak, 1994; Hynes, 1997; McNeil, 1993; Pronk, 1993; White, 1994) as well as rejecting (Coleman, 1995; Harvey, 1987; Moberly, 1983; National Conference of Catholic Bishops, 1982; Nicolosi, 1991; van den Aardweg, 1997) interpretations of homosexuality. Some denominations are more accepting of homosexuality than others, and most are more willing to talk about the subject than they were thirty years ago. While the gay-rejectionist stance among organized religions currently holds greater political power and dictates what passes as today's "correct" interpretations of scripture, the future of their ability to maintain doctrinal sway remains uncertain.[11]

From a psychoanalytic perspective, it seems both unwise and unhelpful for a therapist to unquestioningly endorse one side of a patient's religious conflict. Yet given their stated idealization of institutions that reject homosexuality, not to mention their obvious disdain for relativism, reparative therapists, at least in their published works, do not accept or respect any religious view that affirms homosexuality. Given their wholesale endorsement of heterosexual, social conformity, these therapists seem unable to empathize with conflicted patients who question orthodox or fundamentalist views regarding homosexuality. As the reparative therapy approach precludes the possibility of a deeper investigation into a religiously conflicted patient's full range of feelings about same-sex attractions, it is a clinical stance with troubling ethical implications.

ETHICAL ISSUE I:
REPARATIVE THERAPY AND THE LACK OF RESPECT

Today, reparative therapists argue that patients with same-sex attractions have a mental illness if they believe they suffer from one; they further assert that this illness should be treated. This argument was previously put forward and encoded in the DSM-II as Sexual Orientation Disturbance (American Psychiatric Association, 1968), later changed in the DSM-III to Ego-Dystonic Homosexuality (American Psychiatric Association, 1980) and then deleted from the revised DSM-III-R (American Psychiatric Association, 1987) altogether.[12] Reparative therapists have kept the ego-dystonic homosexuality argument alive and argue that therapists have an ethical obligation to help these conflicted patients find a reparative therapist. As previously noted, some have argued that this should be done out of respect for the patient's religious and/or cultural beliefs (Yarhouse, 1998).

Respect for any patient's religious and cultural beliefs is paramount if treatment is to occur. However, a therapeutic environment should also entail respect for a patient's real and fantasied deviations from conventional beliefs, not to mention the patient's sexual feelings, fantasies and behaviors. This means respect for a patient also means respecting the patient's same-sex attractions. One finds a great lack of respect, however, in reparative therapy's literature which is characterized by gender stereotyping based upon the most rudimentary cultural notions (Drescher, 1998a, b, d). This literature reifies popular gender beliefs such as "It is in man's nature to be a hunter. Women, being essentially nurturing, are born to be mothers." It also reads as a bestiary of antihomosexual stereotypes: "Homosexuals rarely participate in athletics or competitive sports because of childhood fears of being different from other boys" (Socarides, 1968, p. 136). "Some young men [engage in homosexual activity] to advance their careers. Some actors, for example. They have made it into the movies by going to bed with directors or producers who prefer same-sex" (Socarides, 1995, p. 18). "In some homosexuals, their lifestyles are intimately connected with their careers. Some 90 percent of the men in New York's fashion world are homosexuals" (Socarides, 1995, p. 103). Even the technical language of reparative theory cannot disguise its disdain for same-sex relationships:

> There is no empathic affective reciprocity in the male homosexual relationship. Each partner is playing his part as if in isolation with no cognizance of the complementariness of a sexual union, as if the act were consummated in "splendid isolation" with the other person merely a device for the enactment of a unilateral emotional conflict. . . . The imagery accompanying the homosexual act between males is total fantasy without relevance of the other except as a device. This is a masturbatory equivalent and highly narcissistic . . . There is no reality awareness of the partner or his feelings; the contact is simply epidermal, mucous and anatomic . . . The "welfare emotions," those arising from pleasure, are conspicuously absent: joy, love, tenderness, and pride . . . This is the enactment of the fundamental nature of their object relationships: relating to part objects, not whole objects. (Socarides, 1968, pp. 135-136)

Compounding the lack of respect in their literature is the position taken by NARTH when, in 1994, the AMA called for "nonjudgmental recognition of sexual orientation by physicians" with "respect and concern for their [patients'] lives and values" (Hausman, 1995, p. 18). Reparative therapists, through the voice of their official organization, disagreed: "One wonders how reasonable it is for the AMA to mandate respect (rather than simply tolerance) for every person's 'life and values' " (National Association for Research and Treatment of Homosexuality, 1994). Given these open displays of disrespectful antihomosexual biases, it seems unwise to interpret professional, ethical principles as requiring any patient to be referred to reparative therapists.

ETHICAL ISSUE II:
HARM TO PATIENTS

One of medicine's oldest ethical principles is "First, do no harm." A disrespectful treatment modality may pose a significant risk to those individuals with same-sex attractions who do not change and who may eventually adopt a gay identity. Anecdotal clinical accounts of gay male patients who previously tried to therapeutically alter their sexual attractions indicates that they were often traumatized by the reparative therapy experience itself (Duberman, 1991; Isay, 1996; Drescher, 1998d). Mel White writes:

> For the next years, I read and memorized biblical texts on faith. I fasted and prayed for healing. I believed that God had "healed me" or was "in the process of healing me." But over the long haul, my sexual orientation didn't change. My natural attraction to men never lessened. My need for a long-term, loving relationship with another gay man just increased with every prayer.
>
> After months of trying, my psychiatrist implied that I wasn't really cooperating with the Spirit of God. "He is trying to heal you," the doctor said, "but you are hanging on to the old man and not reaching out to the new." After that, my guilt and fear just escalated.
>
> In fact, the doctor was wrong. He had promised me that if I had enough faith, God would completely change my sexual orientation. I was clinging to that promise like a rock climber clings to the face of a cliff. You can imagine how confused and guilt-ridden I became when my homosexuality stayed firmly in place and the new heterosexual man I hoped to become continued to elude me. (White, 1994, p. 107)

Although anecdotal evidence may be insufficient to satisfy scientific demands, those experiences should give reasonable pause to clinicians before referring anyone to a reparative therapist. Furthermore, the American Psychiatric Association (1998) has taken the following position regarding the potentially harmful effects of reparative therapies:

> The potential risks of "reparative therapy" are great, including depression, anxiety and self-destructive behavior, since therapist alignment with societal prejudices against homosexuality may reinforce self-hatred already experienced by the patient. Many patients who have undergone "reparative therapy" relate that they were inaccurately told that homosexuals are lonely, unhappy individuals who never achieve acceptance or satisfaction. The possibility that the person might achieve happiness and satisfying interpersonal relationships as a gay man or lesbian is not presented, nor are alternative approaches to dealing the effects of societal stigmatization discussed.[13]

ETHICAL ISSUE III:
REPARATIVE THERAPY AND SOCIAL CONFORMITY

Reparative therapists often extol the benefits of heterosexual, social conformity and believe a therapist's role is to help patients who seek conformity to achieve that goal:

> Those who seek reparative therapy do not blame social stigma for their
> unhappiness. Many have looked into the gay life-style, have journeyed
> what became for them a "via negativa," and returned disillusioned by
> what they saw. Their definition of self is integrally woven into traditional
> family life. They refuse to relinquish their heterosexual social identity.
> Rather than wage war against the natural order of society, they instead
> take up the sword of an interior struggle. (Nicolosi, 1991, p. 5)

Religious reparative therapists also eschew any treatment approach that
smacks of moral relativism. Yarhouse (1998), for example, criticizes the gay
affirmative psychotherapy literature for helping religious gay patients find
spiritual support outside those religious institutions which condemn homosexuality. Speaking from what he calls "the organized religious perspective," he
accuses those who have spiritual values with which he disagrees of having "an
understanding of religion [which] is truncated and myopic" (p. 251) while he
claims to speak for the "many homosexual persons [who] are committed to
these [organized, antihomosexual religious] institutions, agree with the historical teachings concerning the moral status of same-sex behavior, and seek to
live in conformity with the teachings of their religious community" (p. 251).

Put another way, reparative therapy's religiously-based traditions hold it to
be a therapist's duty to reinforce social expectations for heterosexual normativity. A similar position was taken in the psychoanalytic literature where
Ovesey (1969), thirty years ago, warned that "Those who lack conviction that
homosexuality is a treatable illness, but believe instead that it is a natural constitutional variant, should not accept homosexuals as patients" (p. 119). In
their appeal for social conformity, reparative therapists disdain moral relativism as an unsatisfactory basis for treatment. Nicolosi (1991) writes:

> In the 1960's, the humanistic movement then influenced psychology into
> a new but disguised version of moral authority. Its new reliance was on
> the gauge of feelings to assess morality. This popular movement of the
> sixties and seventies opposed the psychological tradition and preached
> emotional openness, spontaneity, and loyalty to oneself. Growth was no
> longer seen as a product of intelligence and problem-solving, but rather
> was viewed solely in emotional terms. "Feeling good about yourself" be-
> came the litmus test of good behavior, a sort of bastardized moral sense.
> This humanistic psychology rejected much of the rationalism of the psy-
> choanalytic tradition. It introduced instead the soft sentiment of full ac-
> ceptance of the person, as he is, without expectations. (pp. 16-17)

To reiterate, reparative therapy is based upon a treatment philosophy that
abhors the implicit sexual or moral relativism of normal variant theories. A pa-

tient in reparative therapy must adopt conventional values and gender beliefs as an explicit requirement of the treatment. Nicolosi, for example, believes "effective treatment takes its direction from a shared value system between client and therapist" (1991, p. 17).

It would be difficult to find any patient who did not struggle between individualistic and conformistic wishes. Yet, therapists who take the position that they are primarily agents of the patients' wishes for social conformity do so at their patients' risk. Any therapist can either inhibit or permit the emergence of a patient's inner struggles into consciousness. But reparative therapists buttress only one side of the patient's conflict and, in so doing, they appeal to antihomosexual moral values. Some compliant patients can use a therapist's antihomosexual moral stance to suppress same-sex feelings. However, gay men who anecdotally report "successful" reparative therapies, often return to homosexual activity because their inhibitions were not permanent (White, 1994; Isay, 1996). Because inner conflicts are not allowed full expression, a patient may retain forbidden homoerotic desires while the therapist, and perhaps a spouse, a family or a community of faith reinforce the prohibitive role. In suppressing homoerotic desires, the appearance of a heterosexual identity is created and the values of the patient's social order are maintained:

> In my third year of analysis my future wife and I became engaged. My analyst, who had never called me by name in our sessions because he felt it would interfere with the perception of his neutrality, enthusiastically congratulated me. And although he was on vacation at the time, he sent a warm telegram to the synagogue on the occasion of our marriage the following summer. (Isay, 1996, p. 19)

It is certainly worth questioning, on both therapeutic and ethical grounds, whether encouraging conformity over individuality is a valid treatment goal. Should therapists be allowed to question a patient's "autonomous wish" for social conformity or should such wishes simply be taken at face value? These are difficult and important clinical questions, but reparative therapists have not convincingly addressed them.

ETHICAL ISSUE IV: REPARATIVE THERAPY AND INFORMED CONSENT

Nicolosi (1991) says that "Reparative therapy is not a 'cure' in the sense of erasing all homosexual feelings" (p. xviii). Bieber (Bieber et al., 1962) claimed a 27 percent success rate for psychoanalytic conversions of homosexuality while Socarides (1968, 1995) claims a 35 percent conversion rate of the homosexually-identified patients he treated since 1967. Over the last 40 years, the claims made in these reports have never been followed up in any rigorous, scientific way.

Informed consent would require that every potential patient should be given this information before agreeing to undergo a reparative therapy. However, even when informed consent is given, often the circumstances surrounding reparative therapies create unreasonable expectations. Clinical experience has shown that individuals who are desperately attempting to conform to heterosexual normativity are willing to make major sacrifices of time, effort, and money to achieve that goal. Again, anecdotal reports indicate that when the treatment fails, the patient often blames that failure on him or herself. Reparative therapists often claim or imply that the patient's motivation to change primarily determines the success or failure of reparative therapy. This only reinforces feelings of failure and incompetence in those who cannot change. As a result, an unsuccessful outcome can leave an "unrepaired" patient feeling ashamed and depressed, and sometimes in worse condition than when the treatment began.[14]

From a technical standpoint, however, providing a patient with informed consent for reparative therapy can undermine that treatment. For as Mitchell (1981) notes, traditional, analytically-oriented reparative therapies are "exploitations of the transference" which rely upon "directive-suggestive approaches" that evoke a "false-self compliance." Religious reparative therapies, like the faith healing from which they are ultimately derived, are a treatment modality that purports to provide definitive answers regarding human nature and sexuality. They always define homosexuality as morally wrong and require that those individuals trying to change their sexual orientation submit to the therapist's authority as a condition of treatment (Drescher, 1998d). Mitchell further notes that reparative therapists seem "simply unconcerned about the extent to which the approach they urge makes behavioral changes motivated by a compliant transference likely, and the extent to which their own illustrations strongly suggest this possibility" (1981, p. 69). For in reparative therapies, it is the client's compliance with the therapist's authority, rather than the therapist's interpretations, that will determine the outcome of treatment. This too is a clinical stance with troubling ethical implications.

CONCLUSION

To repeat, reparative therapies raise many ethical questions. Reparative therapists have responded to them with claims of immunity: "The contract entered into by analyst and analysand is a private one. Once embarked in a treatment, the goals are the concern of the patient and analyst only . . . " (Socarides et al., 1999). This objection, however, is valid only up to a point. It presumes that the patient and therapist are engaged in a therapeutic activity that would be acceptable to one's professional colleagues and current standards of care. In fact, there exist many limitations on the right of patients and therapists to do anything they wish. These include peer review, laws governing physician-patient relationships, as well as patient complaints to medical licensing boards and professional ethics committees.

The ethical concerns surrounding reparative therapy practices have been discussed here and elsewhere (Haldeman, 1994; Brown, 1996; Drescher, 1997, 1998b). Some of those questions bear repeating: Do reparative therapists routinely tell their potential patients of the two-thirds probability that they won't change? Should they warn patients that if they don't change, they might feel worse about themselves than when they started? Is it ethical for a therapist to offer their professional credentials and opinions in support of criminalizing same-sex behaviors, even when that clinician believes homosexuality is an illness? Should a therapist evaluating or treating a patient in reparative therapy be ethically obliged to tell the patient if he or she has ever testified in favor of sodomy laws? Should informed consent include a therapist volunteering to a prospective client that they support in word, deed or action, laws that criminalize same-sex behaviors? Might one not expect serious ethical problems when a therapist's antihomosexual attitudes and values get played out with patients who enter treatment having been exposed to similar values that have profoundly affected their capacity to accept themselves for who they are? This is a discussion that not only involves reparative therapists and their patients, but anyone concerned about the social, professional, ethical and moral implications of psychotherapy practice.

In closing, it should be noted that a logical extension of the ethical arguments put forward by reparative therapists is that those in the mental health mainstream who respect sexual diversity operate under a different code of ethics than the clinicians who believe homosexuality is immoral or wrong. Will the fundamentally different value systems in the culture wars create contradictory ethical obligations for clinicians? Until recently, mainstream organizations have been unwilling to address this question. Yet if contradictory ethical obligations are emerging in the mental health fields as a result of social changes, this is an important and challenging topic of concern to anyone interested in developing professional standards of conduct and treatment. Open discussion of the subject is something that the leaders in the field owe to our professions and to our patients.

NOTES

1. From The Principles of Medical Ethics with Annotations Especially Applicable to Psychiatry (American Psychiatric Association, 1993). This principle is from Section 1 and goes on to say that "A psychiatrist should not be a party to any type of policy that excludes, segregates, or demeans the dignity of any patient because of ethnic origin,

race, sex, creed, age, socioeconomic status, or *sexual orientation* (p. 3, emphasis added).

2. The author is thankful to Todd Essig, PhD, for this analogy.

3. A developmental arrest (Freud, 1905) was defined as a form of psychological immaturity; not quite an illness, but not quite health either (cf. Drescher, 1996).

4. See Appendix 1.

5. See Appendix 2.

6. The last decade was characterized by an unprecedented public debate about the social status of homosexuality in the military, in the civilian workplace as well as increasing attention regarding the rights of members of same-sex relationships to marry or to raise children (Bawer, 1993; Shilts, 1993; Woods and Lucas, 1993; Eskridge, 1996; Sullivan, 1995, 1997; Group for the Advancement of Psychiatry, 2000).

7. See Appendix 3 for the entire text of this letter.

8. The advertisement read: "Only 8% of homosexual couples report relationships of more than 3 years duration" (NARTH Conference: *Making Sense of Homosexuality,* Claremont Institute, Benjamin Kaufman, MD, Los Angeles, CA, 10/24/98).

9. There is actually a growing social constructivist literature which challenges essentialist claims and yet is also gay-affirming (see, for example, Abelove et al., 1993; Butler, 1993, 1995; Cabaj and Stein, 1996; Chodorow, 1992; Domenici and Lesser, 1995; Magee and Miller, 1997; Schwartz, 1998; Lesser and Schoenberg, 1999).

10. He even suggested several etiological factors leading to homophobia: the religious motive, the secret fear of being homosexual, repressed envy, and the threat to values.

11. See Gomes (1996) for a discussion of a parallel scriptural debate about the religious support for slavery and racism in the ante-bellum United States.

12. See Krajeski (1996) for a more detailed explanation of those events.

13. See Appendix 1 for the full text of the APA Position statement.

14. See Appendix 1.

REFERENCES

Abelove, H., Barale, M.A., & Halperin, D., eds. (1993), *The Lesbian and Gay Studies Reader.* New York: Routledge.

American Psychiatric Association (1968), *Diagnostic and Statistical Manual of Mental Disorders, 2nd Edition.* Washington, DC: American Psychiatric Press.

American Psychiatric Association (1980), *Diagnostic and Statistical Manual of Mental Disorders, 3rd Edition.* Washington, DC: American Psychiatric Press.

American Psychiatric Association (1987), *Diagnostic and Statistical Manual of Mental Disorders, 3rd Edition–Revised.* Washington, DC: American Psychiatric Press.

American Psychiatric Association (1993), *The Principles of Medical Ethics: With Annotations Especially Applicable to Psychiatry.* Washington, DC: American Psychiatric Press.

American Psychiatric Association (1998), *Position Statement on Psychiatric Treatment and Sexual Orientation,* December 11.

American Psychiatric Association (2000), Commission on Psychotherapy by Psychiatrists (COPP): Position statement on therapies focused on attempts to change sexual orientation (Reparative or conversion therapies). *Amer. J. Psychiat.*, 157:1719-1721.

American Psychological Association (1992), Ethical principles of psychologists and code of conduct. *Amer. Psychologist*, 47(12):1597-1611.

Bawer, B. (1993), *A Place at the Table: The Gay Individual in American Society*. New York: Poseidon Press.

Bayer, R. (1981), *Homosexuality and American Psychiatry; The Politics of Diagnosis*. New York: Basic Books.

Bell, A., Weinberg, M., & Hammersmith S. (1981), *Sexual Preference: Its Development in Men and Women*. Bloomington, IN: Indiana University Press.

Blechner, M. (1993), Homophobia in psychoanalytic writing and practice. *Psychoanal. Dial.*, 3:627-637.

Bieber, I., Dain, H., Dince, P., Drellich, M., Grand, H., Gundlach, R., Kremer, M., Rifkin, A., Wilbur, C., & Bieber T. (1962), *Homosexuality: A Psychoanalytic Study*. New York: Basic Books.

Boswell, J. (1980), *Christianity, Social Tolerance and Homosexuality*. Chicago, IL: University of Chicago Press.

Boswell, J. (1994), *Same-Sex Unions in Premodern Europe*. New York: Villard Books.

Brown, L.S. (1996), Ethical concerns with sexual minority patients. In: *Textbook of Homosexuality and Mental Health*. ed. R. Cabaj & T. Stein. Washington, DC: American Psychiatric Press, pp. 897-916.

Bullough, V. (1979), *Homosexuality: A History*. New York: Meridian.

Butler, J. (1993), *Bodies that Matter: On the Discursive Limits of Sex*. New York: Routledge.

Butler, J. (1995), Melancholy gender–Refused identification. *Psychoanal. Dial.*, 5: 165-180.

Byne, W. & Stein, E. (1997), Varieties of Biological Explanation. *The Harvard Gay and Lesbian Review*, Winter, pp. 13-15.

Cabaj, R. & Stein, T., eds. (1996), *Textbook of Homosexuality and Mental Health*. Washington, DC: American Psychiatric Press.

Campbell v. Sundquist (1995), Memorandum and Order, 93C-1547, February 2.

Carrol, W. (1997), On being gay and an American Baptist minister. *The InSpiriter*, Spring, pp. 6-7,11.

Chodorow, N.J. (1992), Heterosexuality as a compromise formation: Reflections on the psychoanalytic theory of sexual development. *Psychoanal. Contemp. Thought*, 15:267-304.

Cohen, R. (1998a), Voir Dire Testimony taken before the Honorable Carolyn Jefferson, Judge, State of Louisiana, Civil District Court for the Parish of Orleans, CDC No. 94-9260, Section 5, Division "A," October 30.

Cohen, R. (1998b), Testimony taken before the Honorable Carolyn Jefferson, Judge, State of Louisiana, Civil District Court for the Parish of Orleans, CDC No. 94-9260, Section 5, Division "A," October 30.

Coleman, G. (1995), *Homosexuality: Catholic Teaching and Pastoral Practice*. Mahwah, NJ: Paulist Press.

DeCecco, J. & Parker, D., eds. (1995), *Sex, Cells and Same-Sex Desire. The Biology of Sexual Preference*. New York: Harrington Park Press.

Domenici, T. & Lesser, R., eds. (1995), *Disorienting Sexuality: Psychoanalytic Reappraisals of Sexual Identities*. New York: Routledge.

Drescher, J. (1996), A discussion across sexual orientation and gender boundaries: Reflections of a gay male analyst to a heterosexual female analyst. *Gender & Psychoanal.*, 1(2):223-237.

Drescher, J. (1997), What needs changing? Some questions raised by reparative therapy practices. *New York State Psychiatric Society Bulletin*, 40(1):8-10.

Drescher, J. (1998a), I'm your handyman: A history of reparative therapies. *J. of Homosexual.*, 36(1):19-42.

Drescher, J. (1998b), Reparative or destructive? Guest Editorial, *Clin. Psychiat. News*, March, p. 12.

Drescher, J. (1998c), Contemporary psychoanalytic psychotherapy with gay men: With a commentary on reparative therapy of homosexuality. *J. of Gay and Lesbian Psychother.*, 2(4):51-74

Drescher, J. (1998d), *Psychoanalytic Therapy and The Gay Man*. Hillsdale, NJ: The Analytic Press.

Dreyfuss, R. (1999), The holy war on gays. *Rolling Stone*, March 18, pp. 38-41.

Duberman, M. (1991), *Cures: A Gay Man's Odyssey*. New York: Dutton.

Eissler, K. (1953), The effect of the structure of the ego on psychoanalytic technique. *J of the Amer. Psychoanal. Assn.*, 1:104-143.

Eskridge, W. (1996), *The Case for Same-Sex Marriage: From Sexual Liberty to Civilized Commitment*. New York: The Free Press.

Ford, C. & Beach, F. (1951), *Patterns of Sexual Behavior*. New York: Harper.

Freud, S. (1905), Three essays on the theory of sexuality. *Standard Edition*, 7:123-246. London: Hogarth Press, 1953.

Freud, S. (1935), Anonymous (Letter to an American mother). In *The Letters of Sigmund Freud*, ed. E. Freud, 1960. New York: Basic Books, pp. 423-424.

Friedman, R.C. & Downey, J. (1995), MacIntosh study faulted. Letter to the editor, *J. Amer. Psychoanal. Assn.*, 43:304-305.

Gadpaille, W. (1989), Homosexuality. In: *Comprehensive Textbook of Psychiatry*, Fifth Edition, eds. H. Kaplan & B. Sadock. Baltimore, MD: Williams and Wilkins, pp. 1086-1096.

Gomes, P.J. (1996), *The Good Book: Reading the Bible with Mind and Heart*. New York: Avon.

Greenberg, D. (1988), *The Construction of Homosexuality*. Chicago, IL: The University of Chicago Press.

Greenhouse, L. (1996), Gay rights laws can't be banned, high court rules: Colorado law void. *The New York Times*, May 21, p. 1.

Group for the Advancement of Psychiatry (2000), *Homosexuality and the Mental Health Professions: The Impact of Bias*. Hillsdale, NJ: The Analytic Press.

Haldeman, D. (1991), Sexual orientation conversion therapy for gay men and lesbians: A scientific examination. In: *Homosexuality: Research Implications for Public Policy*, eds. J. C. Gonsiorek & J. D. Weinrich. Newbury Park, CA: Sage Publications, pp. 149-161.

Haldeman, D. (1994), The practice and ethics of sexual orientation conversion therapy. *J. of Consulting and Clin. Psychol.*, 62(2):221-227.

Harvey, J. (1987), *The Homosexual Person: New Thinking in Pastoral Care*. San Francisco, CA: Ignatius.

Hatterer, L. (1970), *Changing Homosexuality in the Male*. New York: McGraw Hill.

Hausman, K. (1995), AMA reverses stand on homosexual issues. *Psychiat. News*, 30(2), pp. 1,18.

Hausman, K. (2000), APA stakes out positions on controversial therapies. *Psychiat. News*, 34(2), April 21, pp. 45,66.

Helminiak, D. (1994), *What the Bible Really Says About Homosexuality*. San Francisco, CA: Alamo Press.

Hooker, E. (1957), The adjustment of the male overt homosexual. *J. Proj. Tech.*, 21:18-31.

Hynes, W. (1997), Simply home: Integrity/Staten Island finds a seat at the table for lesbians and gays. *Staten Island Advance*, December 13, pp. B1,4.

Isay, R. (1996), *Becoming Gay: The Journey to Self-Acceptance*. New York: Pantheon.

Katz, J. (1995), *The Invention of Heterosexuality*. New York: Dutton.

Kinsey, A., Pomeroy, W., & Martin, C. (1948), *Sexual Behavior in the Human Male*. Philadelphia, PA: Saunders.

Kinsey, A., Pomeroy, W., Martin, C., & Gebhard, P. (1953), *Sexual Behavior in the Human Female*. Philadelphia, PA: Saunders.

Krajeski, J. (1996), Homosexuality and the Mental Health Professions. In: *Textbook of Homosexuality and Mental Health*, ed. R. Cabaj & T. Stein. Washington, DC: American Psychiatric Press, pp. 17-31.

Lesser, R. & Schoenberg, E. (1999), *That Obscure Subject of Desire: Freud's Female Homosexual Revisited*. New York: Routledge.

Lewes, K. (1988), *The Psychoanalytic Theory of Male Homosexuality*. New York: Simon and Schuster. Reissued as *Psychoanalysis and Male Homosexuality* (1995), Northvale, NJ: Aronson.

MacIntosh, H. (1994), Attitudes and experiences of psychoanalysts in analyzing homosexual patients. *J. Amer. Psychoanal. Assn.*, 42:1183-1207.

Magee, M. & Miller, D. (1997), *Lesbian Lives: Psychoanalytic Narratives Old and New*. Hillsdale, NJ: The Analytic Press.

Marmor, J., ed. (1965), *Sexual Inversion: The Multiple Roots of Homosexuality*. New York: Basic Books.

Marmor, J., ed. (1980), *Homosexual Behavior: A Modern Reappraisal*. New York: Basic Books.

McNeil, J. (1993), *The Church and the Homosexual, Fourth Edition*. Boston, MA: Beacon.

McWhirter, D., Sanders, S., & Reinisch, J., eds. (1990), *Homosexuality/Heterosexuality: Concepts of Sexual Orientation*. New York: Oxford University Press.

Mitchell, S. (1981), The psychoanalytic treatment of homosexuality: Some technical considerations. *Int. Rev. Psycho-Anal.*, 8:63-80.

Moberly, E. (1983), *Homosexuality: A New Christian Ethic*. Cambridge, UK: James Clarke & Co.

National Association for Research and Treatment of Homosexuality (1994), New AMA Policy Statement. *NARTH Bulletin*, 2(3), December, p. 5.

National Conference of Catholic Bishops (1982), *Norms for Priestly Formation*. Washington, DC: United States Catholic Conference.

New Hampshire Christian Coalition (1999), It's time to protect New Hampshire's children: Say NO to HB 90. *Manchester Union Leader*, February 1, paid advertisement.

Nicolosi, J. (1991), *Reparative Therapy of Male Homosexuality: A New Clinical Approach*. Northvale, NJ: Aronson.

Nicolosi, J. (2000), Letter to the editor. *Psychiatric News*, 35(3):13,25, February 4.

Ovesey, L. (1969), *Homosexuality and Pseudohomosexuality*. New York: Science House.

Pronk, P. (1993), *Against Nature: Types of Moral Argumentation Regarding Homosexuality*. Grand Rapids, MI: William B. Eerdmans.

Rado, S. (1940), A critical examination of the concept of bisexuality. *Psychosomatic Medicine*, 2:459-467. Reprinted in *Sexual Inversion: The Multiple Roots of Homosexuality*, ed. J. Marmor. New York: Basic Books, 1965, pp. 175-189.

Rado, S. (1969), *Adaptational Psychodynamics: Motivation and Control*. New York: Science House.

Roughton, R. (1995), Overcoming antihomosexual bias: A progress report. *The American Psychoanalyst*, 29(4):15-16.

Schwartz, A. (1998), *Sexual Subjects: Lesbians, Gender, and Psychoanalysis*. New York: Routledge.

Schwartz, D. (1993), Heterophilia–The love that dare not speak its aim. *Psychoanal. Dial.*, 3:643-652.

Shilts, R. (1993), *Conduct Unbecoming: Gays and Lesbians in the U.S. Military*. New York: St. Martin's Press.

Siegel, E. (1988), *Female Homosexuality: Choice Without Volition*. Hillsdale, NJ: The Analytic Press.

Socarides, C. (1968), *The Overt Homosexual*. New York: Grune & Stratton.

Socarides, C. (1978), *Homosexuality*. New York: Jason Aronson.

Socarides, C. (1993), District Court, City and County of Denver, Colorado. Case No. 92 CV 7223. Affidavit of Charles W. Socarides, M.D. *Evans. v. Romer*.

Socarides, C. (1994a), Response to Judd Marmor, M.D. *Psychiatric News*, May 20.

Socarides, C. (1994b), The erosion of heterosexuality. *The Washington Times*, July 5.

Socarides, C. (1995), *Homosexuality: A Freedom Too Far*. Phoenix, AZ: Adam Margrave Books.

Socarides, C., Kaufman, B., Nicolosi, J., Satinover, J., & Fitzgibbons, R. (1997), Don't forsake homosexuals who want help. *The Wall Street Journal*, January 9.

Socarides, C., Freedman, A., Tait, C., Kaufman, B., & Voth, H. (1999), Reparative Therapy. Letter to the Editor, *Psychiat. News*, April 16, pp. 41,50.

Sullivan, A. (1995), *Virtually Normal: An Argument About Homosexuality*. New York: Knopf.

Sullivan, A., ed. (1997), *Same-Sex Marriage: Pro and Con*. New York: Vintage Books.

Szasz, T. (1974), *Ceremonial Chemistry*. New York: Anchor Books.

Tiffen, L. (1994), *Creationism's Upside-Down Pyramid: How Science Refutes Fundamentalism*. Amherst, NY: Prometheus Books.

Trop, J. & Stolorow, R. (1993), Reply to Blechner, Lesser, and Schwartz. *Psychoanal. Dial.*, 2:653-656.

van den Aardweg, G. (1997), *The Battle for Normality: A Guide for (Self-) Therapy for Homosexuality*. San Francisco, CA: Ignatius Press.

Weinberg, G. (1972), *Society and the Healthy Homosexual*. New York: Anchor Books.

White, M. (1994), *Stranger at the Gate: To Be Gay and Christian in America*. New York: Simon & Schuster.

Woods, J. & Lucas, J. (1993), *The Corporate Closet: The Professional Lives of Gay Men in America*. New York: The Free Press.

Yarhouse, M. (1998), When clients seek treatment for same-sex attraction: Ethical issues in the "Right to Choose" debate. *Psychotherapy: Theory/Research/Practice/Training*, 35(2):248-259.

Zwillich, T. (1999), APA formally rejects curing homosexuals. *Clin. Psychiat, News*, January, p. 5.

APPENDIX 1

American Psychiatric Association Position Statement
on Psychiatric Treatment and Sexual Orientation
December 11, 1998

The Board of Trustees of the American Psychiatric Association removed homosexuality from the DSM in 1973 after reviewing evidence that is was not a mental disorder. In 1987, ego-dystonic homosexuality was not included in the DSM-III-R after a similar review.

The American Psychiatric Association does not currently have a formal position statement on treatments that attempt to change a person's sexual orientation, also known as "reparative or conversion therapy." There is an APA 1997 Fact Sheet on Homosexual and Bisexual Issues which states that "there is no published scientific evidence supporting the efficacy of 'reparative therapy' as a treatment to change one's sexual orientation."

The potential risks of "reparative therapy" are great, including depression, anxiety and self-destructive behavior, since therapist alignment with societal prejudices against homosexuality may reinforce self-hatred already experienced by the patient. Many patients who have undergone "reparative therapy" relate that they were inaccurately told that homosexuals are lonely, unhappy individuals who never achieve acceptance or satisfaction. The possibility that the person might achieve happiness and satisfying interpersonal relationships as a gay man or lesbian is not presented, nor are alternative approaches to dealing with the effects of societal stigmatization discussed. The APA recognizes that in the course of ongoing psychiatric treatment there may be appropriate clinical indications for attempting to change sexual behaviors.

Several major professional organizations including the American Psychological Association, the National Association of Social Workers and the American Academy of Pediatrics have all made statements against "reparative therapy" because of concerns for the harm caused to patients. The American Psychiatric Association has already taken clear stands against discrimination, prejudice and unethical treatment on a variety of issues including discrimination on the basis of sexual orientation.

Therefore, the American Psychiatric Association opposes any psychiatric treatment, such as "reparative" or "conversion" therapy which is based upon the assumption that homosexuality per se is a mental disorder or based upon the a priori assumption that the patient should change his/her sexual homosexual orientation.

APPENDIX 2

American Psychiatric Association
Commission on Psychotherapy by Psychiatrists (COPP)
Position Statement on Therapies Focused on Attempts to Change Sexual
Orientation (Reparative or Conversion Therapies)

PREAMBLE

In December of 1998, the Board of Trustees issued a position statement that the American Psychiatric Association opposes any psychiatric treatment, such as "reparative" or conversion therapy, which is based upon the assumption that homosexuality per se is a mental disorder or based upon the a priori assumption that a patient should change his/her sexual homosexual orientation (Appendix 1). In doing so, the APA joined many other professional organizations that either oppose or are critical of "reparative" therapies, including the American Academy of Pediatrics, the American Medical Association, the American Psychological Association, The American Counseling Association, and the National Association of Social Workers.[1]

The following Position Statement expands and elaborates upon the statement issued by the Board of Trustees in order to further address public and professional concerns about therapies designed to change a patient's sexual orientation or sexual identity. It augments rather than replaces the 1998 statement.

POSITION STATEMENT

In the past, defining homosexuality as an illness buttressed society's moral opprobrium of same-sex relationships.[2] In the current social climate, claiming homosexuality is a mental disorder stems from efforts to discredit the growing social acceptance of homosexuality as a normal variant of human sexuality. Consequently, the issue of changing sexual orientation has become highly politicized. The integration of gays and lesbians into the mainstream of American society is opposed by those who fear that such an integration is morally wrong and harmful to the social fabric. The political and moral debates surrounding this issue have obscured the scientific data by calling into question the motives and even the character of individuals on both sides of the issue. This document attempts to shed some light on this heated issue.

The validity, efficacy and ethics of clinical attempts to change an individual's sexual orientation have been challenged.[3,4,5,6] To date, there are no scientifically rigorous outcome studies to determine either the actual efficacy or harm of reparative treatments. There is sparse scientific data about selection criteria, risks versus benefits of the treatment, and long-term outcomes of reparative therapies. The literature consists of anecdotal reports of individuals who have claimed to change, people who claim that attempts to change were harmful to them, and others who claimed to have changed and then later recanted those claims.[7,8,9]

With little data about patients, it is possible to evaluate the theories which rationalize the conduct of "reparative" or conversion therapies. Firstly, they are at odds with the scientific position of the American Psychiatric Association which has maintained, since 1973, that homosexuality per se, is not a mental disorder. The theories of "reparative" therapists define homosexuality as either a developmental arrest, a severe form of psychopathology, or some combination of both.[10-15] In recent years, noted practitioners of "reparative therapy" have openly integrated older psychoanalytic theories that pathologize homosexuality with traditional religious beliefs condemning homosexuality.[16,17,18]

The earliest scientific criticisms of the early theories and religious beliefs informing "reparative" or conversion therapies came primarily from sexology researchers.[19-27] Later, criticisms emerged from psychoanalytic sources as well.[28-39] There has also been an increasing body of religious thought arguing against traditional, biblical interpretations that condemn homosexuality and which underlie religious types of "reparative" therapy.[40-46]

RECOMMENDATIONS

1. APA affirms its 1973 position that homosexuality per se is not a diagnosable mental disorder. Recent publicized efforts to repathologize homosexuality by claiming that it can be cured are often guided not by

rigorous scientific or psychiatric research, but sometimes by religious and political forces opposed to a full civil rights for gay men and lesbians. APA recommends that the APA respond quickly and appropriately as a scientific organization when claims that homosexuality is a curable illness are made by political or religious groups.

2. As a general principle, a therapist should not determine the goal of treatment either coercively or through subtle influence. Psychotherapeutic modalities to convert or "repair" homosexuality are based on developmental theories whose scientific validity is questionable. Furthermore, anecdotal reports of "cures" are counterbalanced by anecdotal claims of psychological harm. In the last four decades, "reparative" therapists have not produced any rigorous scientific research to substantiate their claims of cure. Until there is such research available, APA recommends that ethical practitioners refrain from attempts to change individuals' sexual orientation, keeping in mind the medical dictum to First, do no harm.

3. The "reparative" therapy literature uses theories that make it difficult to formulate scientific selection criteria for their treatment modality. This literature not only ignores the impact of social stigma in motivating efforts to cure homosexuality, it is a literature that actively stigmatizes homosexuality as well. "Reparative" therapy literature also tends to overstate the treatment's accomplishments while neglecting any potential risks to patients. APA encourages and supports research in the NIMH and the academic research community to further determine "reparative" therapy's risks versus its benefits.

REFERENCES

1. National Association for Research and Treatment of Homosexuality, (1999), American Counseling Association Passes Resolution to Oppose Reparative Therapy. NARTH Website (http://www.narth.com/docs/acaresolution.html).

2. Bayer, R. (1981), Homosexuality and American Psychiatry; The Politics of Diagnosis. New York: Basic Books.

3. Haldeman, D. (1991), Sexual orientation conversion therapy for gay men and lesbians: A scientific examination. In Homosexuality: Research Implications for Public Policy, ed. J. C. Gonsiorek & J. D. Weinrich. Newbury Park, CA: Sage Publications, pp. 149-161.

4. Haldeman, D. (1994), The practice and ethics of sexual orientation conversion therapy. J. of Consulting and Clin. Psychol., 62(2):221-227.

5. Brown, L. S. (1996), Ethical concerns with sexual minority patients. In: Textbook of Homosexuality and Mental Health. ed. R. Cabaj & T. Stein. Washington, D.C.: American Psychiatric Press, pp. 897-916.

6. Drescher, J. (1997), What needs changing? Some questions raised by reparative therapy practices. New York State Psychiatric Society Bulletin, 40(1):8-10.

7. Duberman, M. (1991), Cures: A Gay Man's Odyssey. New York: Dutton.

8. White, M. (1994), Stranger at the Gate: To Be Gay and Christian in America. New York: Simon & Schuster.

9. Isay, R. (1996), Becoming Gay: The Journey to Self-Acceptance. New York: Pantheon.

10. Freud, S. (1905), Three Essays on the Theory of Sexuality. Standard Edition, 7:123-246. London: Hogarth Press, 1953.

11. Rado, S. (1940), A critical examination of the concept of bisexuality. Psychosomatic Medicine, 2:459-467. Reprinted in Sexual Inversion: The Multiple Roots of Homosexuality, ed. J. Marmor. New York: Basic Books, 1965, pp. 175-189.

12. Bieber, I., Dain, H., Dince, P., Drellich, M., Grand, H., Gundlach, R., Kremer, M., Rifkin, A., Wilbur, C., & Bieber T. (1962), Homosexuality: A Psychoanalytic Study. New York: Basic Books.

13. Socarides, C. (1968), The Overt Homosexual. New York: Grune & Stratton.

14. Ovesey, L. (1969), Homosexuality and Pseudohomosexuality. New York: Science House.

15. Hatterer, L. (1970), Changing Homosexuality in the Male. New York: McGraw Hill.

16. Moberly, E. (1983), Homosexuality: A New Christian Ethic. Cambridge, UK: James Clarke & Co.

17. Harvey, J. (1987), The Homosexual Person: New Thinking in Pastoral Care. San Francisco, CA: Ignatius.

18. Nicolosi, J. (1991), Reparative Therapy of Male Homosexuality: A New Clinical Approach. Northvale, NJ: Aronson.

19. Kinsey, A., Pomeroy, W., & Martin, C. (1948), Sexual Behavior in the Human Male. Philadelphia, PA: Saunders.

20. Kinsey, A., Pomeroy, W., & Martin, C. and Gebhard, P. (1953), Sexual Behavior in the Human Female. Philadelphia, PA: Saunders.

21. Ford, C. & Beach, F. (1951), Patterns of Sexual Behavior. New York: Harper.

22. Hooker, E. (1957), The adjustment of the male overt homosexual. J. Proj. Tech., 21:18-31.

23. Bell, A. & Weinberg, M. (1978), Homosexualities: A Study of Diversity Among Men and Women. New York: Simon and Schuster.

24. Bell, A., Weinberg, M. & Hammersmith S. (1981), Sexual Preference: Its Development in Men and Women. Bloomington, IN: Indiana University Press.

25. LeVay, S. (1991), A difference in hypothalamic structure between heterosexual and homosexual men. Science, 253:1034-1037.

26. Hamer, D., Hu, S., Magnuson, V., Hu, N. & Pattatucci, A. (1993), A linkage between DNA markers on the X-chromosome and male sexual orientation. Science, 261:321-327.

27. Bem, D. (1996), Exotic becomes erotic: A developmental theory of sexual orientation. Psychol. Review, 103(2):320-335.

28. Marmor, J., ed. (1965), Sexual Inversion: The Multiple Roots of Homosexuality. New York: Basic Books.

29. Mitchell, S. (1978), Psychodynamics, homosexuality, and the question of pathology. Psychiatry, 41:254-263.

30. Marmor, J., ed. (1980), Homosexual Behavior: A Modern Reappraisal. New York: Basic Books.

31. Mitchell, S. (1981), The psychoanalytic treatment of homosexuality: Some technical considerations. Int. Rev. Psycho-Anal., 8:63-80.

32. Morgenthaler, F. (1984), Homosexuality Heterosexuality Perversion, trans. A. Aebi. Hillsdale, NJ: The Analytic Press, 1988.

33. Lewes, K. (1988), The Psychoanalytic Theory of Male Homosexuality. New York: Simon and Schuster. Reissued as Psychoanalysis and Male Homosexuality (1995), Northvale, NJ: Aronson.

34. Friedman, R.C. (1988), Male Homosexuality: A Contemporary Psychoanalytic Perspective. New Haven, CT: Yale University Press.

35. Isay, R. (1989), Being Homosexual: Gay Men and Their Development. New York: Farrar, Straus and Giroux.

36. O'Connor, N. & Ryan, J. (1993), Wild Desires and Mistaken Identities: Lesbianism & Psychoanalysis. New York: Columbia University.

37. Domenici, T. & Lesser, R., eds. (1995) Disorienting Sexuality: Psychoanalytic Reappraisals of Sexual Identities. New York: Routledge.

38. Magee, M. & Miller, D. (1997), Lesbian Lives: Psychoanalytic Narratives Old and New. Hillsdale, NJ: The Analytic Press.

39. Drescher, J. (1998) Psychoanalytic Therapy and The Gay Man. Hillsdale, NJ: The Analytic Press.

40. Boswell, J. (1980), Christianity, Social Tolerance and Homosexuality. Chicago, IL: University of Chicago Press.

41. McNeil, J. (1993), The Church and the Homosexual, Fourth Edition. Boston, MA: Beacon.

42. Pronk, P. (1993), Against Nature: Types of Moral Argumentation Regarding Homosexuality. Grand Rapids, MI: William B. Eerdmans.

43. Boswell, J. (1994), Same-Sex Unions in Premodern Europe. New York: Villard Books.

44. Helminiak, D. (1994), What the Bible Really Says About Homosexuality. San Francisco, CA: Alamo Press.

45. Gomes, P. J. (1996). The Good Book: Reading the Bible with Mind and Heart. New York: Avon.

46. Carrol, W. (1997), On being gay and an American Baptist minister. The InSpiriter, Spring, pp. 6-7,11.

APPENDIX 3

Letter to the Editor
Psychiatric News, Volume 34, Number 3, February 4, 2000
(Reprinted with permission of *Psychiatric News.*)

HOMOSEXUALITY

This is in response to the letter by Jack Drescher, M.D., in the July 2, 2000, issue on reparative therapy. In that letter, Dr. Drescher states, "Some reparative therapists themselves practice sexual politics, albeit on the side opposing gay and lesbian civil rights." He goes on to state that "some reparative therapists endorse criminalizing homosexuality. . . ."

As executive director of the National Association for Research and Therapy of Homosexuality (NARTH), the nation's only professional association dedicated solely to the research and treatment of homosexuality (sometimes known as "reparative therapy"), I would like point out that NARTH does not believe that homosexual practice should be criminalized. Nor do we support the retention of antisodomy laws. Furthermore, the view that homosexuality is a developmental disorder and treatable condition should not be equated with "being against the civil rights of homosexuals."

Legal cases now in the courts do not concern whether gays should be stripped of their civil rights or should have them. The issue is much more complicated: it typically concerns the way the civil-rights laws will be interpreted. Is it just and fair to set up special quota systems to ensure a certain proportion of gays in government job settings? Do homosexuals experience such economic disadvantage that they should be singled out as a protected class of citizens? Saying "no" to such interpretations of the civil-rights laws does not mean that one is "against the civil rights of homosexuals."

Furthermore, there is the larger question as to whether, in general, the law should legitimatize homosexuality on a par with heterosexuality. Our laws cannot be neutral on these issues; the law must inevitably decide (indeed, as it has always done) whether to tolerate or to affirm certain behaviors and lifestyles. When we legitimize gay marriage and adoption and decide (in spite of the overwhelming evidence) that all types of family forms are equally vital to the health of the community and therefore should be given legal recognition, aren't we making foolish decisions that will negatively impact our communal life?

We believe harm would be done if our laws were to affirm homosexuality as indistinguishable from heterosexuality. Children would be adopted by gay couples, whose households are by definition irrevocably motherless or fatherless; greater numbers of sexually confused youth would be encouraged to assume gay identities; we would be forced to teach homosexuality as normative in the public schools; and there would be a further erosion of the nuclear family as the foundation of society.

Gay psychiatrists readily offer the courts their own views, and the national psychological and psychiatric associations take positions on a host of controversial social issues that relate to pending legal cases. We believe it is NARTH's responsibility to counter gay-activist testimony with our perspective, which gay activists call "heterosexist," but which has long served as a foundation of Western civilization and cannot be discarded with mere impunity.

Joseph Nicolosi, PhD
Executive Director
NARTH

Index

Acceptance, desire for, 72-73
Adaptational psychodynamics, 11-12
Amendment Two (Colorado), 188
American Academy of Pediatrics, 91
American Counseling Association, 91,132
American Medical Association, 91
American Psychiatric Association, 91,118,132,169,185
  position statement on changing sexual orientation of, 204-206
  position statement on psychiatric treatment and sexual orientation of, 203-204
  removal of homosexuality from diagnostic nomenclature, 186-187
  reparative therapies and, 185
  representation of homosexuality position of, in conversion therapies, 140-141
American Psychoanalytic Association, 187-188
American Psychological Association, 91,118,132,187-188
  Ethics Code of, 133-134
  representation of homosexuality position of, in conversion therapies, 140-141
  sexual reorientation therapy and, 91
Aversion therapies, 6,77,141,149. *See also* Electric shock therapy

Bayer, R., 186-187

Beckstead, A. Lee, 3,87-115
Behavior therapy, 148-150
Bieber, Irving, 2,12-13,25-34,185,195
Bisexuality, theory of libidinal, 11

Church of Jesus Christ of Latter-day Saints, 94,143
Civil rights, gay, 188
Code of Ethics, for American Psychological Association, 133-134
Coercion
  to remain in conversion therapy, 156-157
  in therapy, 152-153
Cognitive-behavior therapy, 148-150
Community, sense of, and ex-gay movement, 84-85
Confidentiality, violations of, 153-154
Conformity, reparative therapies and, 193-195
Conversion therapies, 2. *See also* Reparative therapies
  agendas for, 88-89
  American Psychiatric Association's Position Statement on, 204-206
  case study of benefits of, 93-106
  coercion to remain in conversion therapy, 156-157
  criticisms of, 132
  current approaches to, 88-89
  de-masculization and, 125-126
  efficacy of, 91
  electric shock treatments, 124

ethical precepts and, 174-178
ethics and, 89-91,133-134
female homosexuality and, 88
informed consent in, 140
male bonding activities and,
    125-126
misinformation during, 140-145
negative side-effects of, 160-162
post, 126
potential harms of, 118-120
proponents of, 132-133
religious/spiritual beliefs and,
    126-127,155-156,159-160
at religious universities, 152-155
vs. reparative therapy, 119-120
representation of APA's positions
    on homosexuality in,
    139-140
research on ethics of, 173-174
self-determination and, 89-91
sexual dysfunction and, 124-125
spirituality and, 126-127
success rates of, 119
termination of, 156
Conversion therapists. *See* Therapists
Cook, Colin, 80-81
Covert sensitization therapy, 78
Cults, 72-73
Culture wars
homosexuality and, 185-187
NARTH and, 188-189
Cures, hoping for, 105-106

Deliverance experiences, 79-80,81
De-masculization, 125-126
Demons, role of, in reparative
    therapies, 79
Depression
risk for, 74
Depression, and loss, 120-122
*Diagnostic and Statistical Manual
    (DSM)*, 169-170
Drescher, Jack, 1-4, 5-22,181-210
Duberman, Martin, 3,37-50,184-185

Early childhood development, Freud's
    theory of, 9
Electric shock therapy, 77,124,168.
    See also Aversion therapies
Emancipation, 83-84
Essentialist view of homosexuality,
    189
Ethical interventions, guidelines for,
    177-178
Ethics
code of, for American
    Psychological Association,
    133-134
conversion therapies and, 174-178
informed consent and, 159
methodology for studying, 134-139
sexual orientation research and,
    173-174
sexual reorientation therapies and,
    89-91
Evergreen International, 100-101
Ex-gay movement, 72-73,91-92
community and, 84-85
counselor training and, 81-82
friendships and, 84-85
political aspects of, 85
sin and, 79
Ex-gay strugglers, 74-75,84-85
Ex-gay theology, 72
martyrdom and, 73
responsibility and, 74
Ex-gay therapy. *See* Reparative
    therapies
Exodus International, 92
Exorcisms, 79-80,81

Female homosexuality, reparative
    therapy and, 88
"First, do no harm." principle, and
    reparative therapies, 192-193
Ford, Jeffrey G., 3,69-86
Forstein, Marshall, 4,167-179
Freud, Sigmund, 2,108,184
on homosexuality, 7-10

theory of early childhood development of, 9
Fundamentalists, 169
  central beliefs of, 72
  ex-gays and, 84
  reparative therapy and, 71-72

Gay civil rights, 188
Gay identity development, model of, 122
  final stage, 127
  second stage, 124
Gilded Age of reparative therapies, 11

Haldeman, Douglas, 3-4
Hatterer, L., 185
Heterosexual bias, 90-91
Heterosexuality, 18-19
  ex-gay view of, 80
Hirschfeld, Magnus, 8,108
Homophobia, 190
Homosexuality
  Bieber's study of, 12-13
  culture wars and, 185-187
  as disorder, 169-170
  essentialist view of, 189
  Freud's theories of, 7-10
  fundamentalists and, 169
  historical perspective of, 184-185
  nature/nurture debate on, 189
  Ovesey's theory of, 14-15
  psychopathological view of, 168
  Rado's theory of, 11-12,15
  removal from diagnostic nomenclature by American Psychiatric Association, 186-187
  sin of, 79
  Socarides's theory of, 13-14
Homosexuals Anonymous, 80
Hooker, Evelyn, 169
Houck, Dough, 82

Informed consent
  accurate information for interventions and prognosis, 145-151
  ethics and, 159
  reparative therapies and, 140,159, 195-196
Inner healing, 81
Intimacy avoidance, 122-124
Isay, Richard, 3,51-67

Kardiner, A., 17-18
Kessler, David, 64-65
Kinney, Robbie, 82
Kinsey, Alfred C., 29
Kinship, 80
Kramer, Larry, 64

Lawson, Ronald, 80
Lesbianism, 88
LGB-affirmative therapists, 107-108
Libidinal bisexuality, theory of, 11
Libido, Freud's psychosexual stages of, 9
Loss, depression and, 120-122

Male bonding, 125-126
Male identity, 125-126
Martyrdom, and ex-gay theology, 73,84
Medical treatments, 175-176
Mental health organizations, culture wars and, 187
Misinformation, during conversion therapies, 140-145
Moberly, Elizabeth, 71,82-83,88,185
Moor, Paul, 2-3,25-36
Moral relativism, 194
Mormons, 94

National Association for Research and
Therapy of Homosexuality
(NARTH), 20-21,145,147,
153,188-189,192,209-210
National Association of Social
Workers, 91,187-188
Nature/nurture debate, of
homosexuality, 189
Nicolosi, J., 17-19,88,145,185,189,
190,194,195,209-210

Ovesey, L., 14-15,185,194

Patients, rights of, 132-133
Paulk, Anne, 92
Paulk, John, 92
Payne, Leanne, 81-82
Peck, M. Scott, 83
Political activism, and reparative
therapists, 187-189
Post-conversion therapies, 126
Prayer therapy, 81
Psychoanalysis, 6-7,11,168-169
Psychoanalytic theory
antihomosexual bias of, 6-7
Psychodynamic therapies, 150
Psychosurgery, 6
Psychotherapy, 185-186
religion-based, 150-151
religious beliefs and, 89-90

Rado, Sandor, 11-12,15,185
Religion
agendas of, 96-97
conversion therapies and,
126-127,155-156,159-160
critical issues in, and conversion
therapies, 159-160
homosexuality and, 190-191
Religion-based psychotherapy,
89-90,150-151

Religious beliefs, psychotherapy and,
89-90
Religious reparative therapies. *See*
Conversion therapies;
Reparative therapies
Religious universities
clinicians at, 154-155
coercion by, 152-153
Reparative therapies, 88. *See also*
Conversion therapies
American Psychiatric Association's
Position Statement on,
204-206
benefits of, 93-94
case study of, 94-106
contemporary, 15-16
conversion rates of, 185
vs. conversion therapies, 119-120
ethical concerns of, 191-197
female homosexuality and, 88
"First, do no harm." principle and,
192-193
fundamentalists and, 71-72
Gilded Age of, 11
historical perspective of, 185
history of, 6,71
informed consent and, 195-196
lack of respect and, 191-192
limitations of, 108-109
moral relativism and, 194
nature/nurture debate and, 189-191
Nicolosi and, 18-19
potential harms of, 118-120
potential risks of, 193
religion and, 72
religious sects and, 72
role of "demons" in, 79
social conformity and, 193-195
success rates of, 119
youths and, 72-73
Reparative therapists. *See* Therapists
Respect, lack of, and reparative
therapies, 191-192
Rundle, Frank, 64-65

Schroeder, Michael, 1-4,131-166
Secret sin, 79
Sects, 72-73
Self-destruction, risk of, 74
Self-determination, of patients, 89-91
Sexual dysfunction, 124-125
Sexual orientation
    American Psychiatric Association's
        position statement on,
        203-204
    changing, 92-93
    changing, with psychotherapy,
        168-170
    current knowledge of, 170-171
    determinants of, 108-109
    ethical issues about research on,
        173-174
    research concerns about, 171-173
    research questions about, 173
Sexual reorientation investigations
    political implications of, 110-111
    research implications of, 110
Sexual reorientation therapies. *See*
        Conversion therapies;
        Reparative therapies
Sexual reorientation therapists. *See*
        Therapists
Shidlo, Ariel, 1-4,131-166
Side-effects, conversion therapy and,
        160-162

Siegel, Elaine, 16-17,88,185
Sin, ex-gay movement and, 79
Socarides, C.,
        13-14,16,19-20,185,192,195
Social conformity, reparative therapies
        and, 193-195
Sodomy laws, 186,188
Spirituality, conversion therapies and,
        126-127. *See also* Religion
Success rates, for conversion therapies,
        119
Suicidal clients, 122

Terminations
    of conversion therapies, 156
    counseling for, 160
    failure to prepare for, 157-158
Therapists
    ethical responsibilities of, 177-178
    issues for contemporary, 15-16
    as political activists, 187-189
    religious, 194
    religious views of, 191
    view of homosexuality by, 191-192
Tripp, C. A., 31-32

Weinberg, George, 190
White, Mel, 193